Pharmacologic Approaches to Heart Failure

Editor

KIRKWOOD F. ADAMS Jr

HEART FAILURE CLINICS

www.heartfailure.theclinics.com

Consulting Editors

MANDEEP R. MEHRA
JAVED BUTLER

October 2014 • Volume 10 • Number 4

ELSEVIER

1600 John F. Kennedy Boulevard • Suite 1800 • Philadelphia, Pennsylvania, 19103-2899

http://www.theclinics.com

HEART FAILURE CLINICS Volume 10, Number 4
October 2014 ISSN 1551-7136, ISBN-13: 978-0-323-32611-7

Editor: Adrianne Brigido
Developmental Editor: Susan Showalter

Heart Failure Clinics (ISSN 1551-7136) is published quarterly by Elsevier Inc., 360 Park Avenue South, New York, NY 10010-1710. Months of publication are January, April, July, and October. Business and editorial offices: 1600 John F. Kennedy Boulevard, Suite 1800, Philadelphia, PA 19103-2899. Periodicals postage paid at New York, NY, and additional mailing offices. Subscription prices are USD 235.00 per year for US individuals, USD 382.00 per year for US institutions, USD 80.00 per year for US students and residents, USD 280.00 per year for Canadian individuals, USD 442.00 per year for Canadian institutions, USD 300.00 per year for international individuals, USD 442.00 per year for international institutions, and USD 100.00 per year for Canadian and foreign students/residents. To receive student and resident rate, orders must be accompanied by name of affiliated institution, date of term, and the *signature* of program/residency coordinator on institution letterhead. Orders will be billed at individual rate until proof of status is received. Foreign air speed delivery is included in all *Clinics* subscription prices. All prices are subject to change without notice. **POSTMASTER:** Send address changes to *Heart Failure Clinics*, Elsevier Health Sciences Division, Subscription Customer Service, 3251 Riverport Lane, Maryland Heights, MO 63043. **Customer Service: 1-800-654-2452 (US and Canada). From outside of the US and Canada, call 314-447-8871. Fax: 314-447-8029. For print support, E-mail: JournalsCustomerService-usa@elsevier.com. For online support, E-mail: JournalsOnlineSupport-usa@elsevier.com.**

Reprints. For copies of 100 or more of articles in this publication, please contact the Commercial Reprints Department, Elsevier Inc., 360 Park Avenue South, New York, NY 10010-1710. Tel.: 212-633-3874; Fax: 212-633-3820; E-mail: reprints@elsevier.com.

Heart Failure Clinics is covered in *MEDLINE/PubMed (Index Medicus)*.

Contributors

CONSULTING EDITORS

MANDEEP R. MEHRA, MD
Co-Director, BWH Heart and Vascular Center;
Executive Director, Center for Advanced Heart
Disease, Brigham and Women's Hospital;
Professor of Medicine, Harvard Medical
School, Boston, Massachusetts

JAVED BUTLER, MD, MPH
Professor of Medicine; Director, Heart Failure
Research, Division of Cardiology, Emory
Clinical Cardiovascular Research Institute,
Emory University, Atlanta, Georgia

EDITOR

KIRKWOOD F. ADAMS Jr, MD
Associate Professor of Medicine/Radiology and
Research Associate Professor of Pharmacy,
Division of Cardiology, UNC Heart and
Vascular, The University of North Carolina
(UNC) at Chapel Hill, Chapel Hill, North Carolina

AUTHORS

KIRKWOOD F. ADAMS Jr, MD
Associate Professor of Medicine/Radiology
and Research Associate Professor of
Pharmacy, Division of Cardiology, UNC Heart
and Vascular, The University of North Carolina
(UNC) at Chapel Hill, Chapel Hill, North Carolina

TARIQ AHMAD, MD, MPH
Division of Cardiology, Duke University
Medical Center; Duke Clinical Research
Institute, Durham, North Carolina

WEERANUN D. BODE, MD
Clinical Fellow, UNC Heart and Vascular
Center, Chapel Hill, North Carolina

JAVED BUTLER, MD, MPH
Professor of Medicine; Director, Heart Failure
Research, Division of Cardiology, Emory
Clinical Cardiovascular Research Institute,
Emory University, Atlanta, Georgia

PATRICIA P. CHANG, MD, MHS
Associate Professor of Medicine; Director,
Heart Failure and Transplant Program, Division
of Cardiology, Department of Medicine, The
University of North Carolina at Chapel Hill,
Chapel Hill, North Carolina

ANDREW CLARK, MD, MA, FRCP
Department of Cardiology, Hull York
Medical School, Castle Hill Hospital,
Kingston-upon-Hull, United Kingdom

**JOHN G.F. CLELAND, MD, PhD, FRCP,
FESC, FACC**
National Heart and Lung Institute, Royal
Brompton and Harefield Hospitals, Imperial
College, London, United Kingdom

ROBERT T. COLE, MD
Division of Cardiology, Emory University,
Atlanta, Georgia

EMILIA D'ELIA, MD
Cardiovascular Department, Papa Giovanni
XXIII Hospital, Bergamo, Italy; University of
Pavia, Pavia, Italy

MONA FIUZAT, PharmD
Division of Cardiology, Duke University
Medical Center; Duke Clinical Research
Institute, Durham, North Carolina

ANIL K. GEHI, MD
Assistant Professor, Electrophysiology,
UNC Heart and Vascular Center, Chapel Hill,
North Carolina

DIVYA GUPTA, MD
Division of Cardiology, Emory University, Atlanta, Georgia

KATE HUTCHINSON, MBChB
Department of Cardiology, Hull York Medical School, Castle Hill Hospital, Kingston-upon-Hull, United Kingdom

BRIAN C. JENSEN, MD
Division of Cardiology, McAllister Heart Institute, University of North Carolina School of Medicine, Chapel Hill, North Carolina

JASON N. KATZ, MD, MHS
Assistant Professor of Medicine; Medical Director, UNC Mechanical Heart Program, Cardiac Intensive Care Unit, and Cardiothoracic Surgical Intensive Care Unit & Critical Care Service; Division of Cardiology, Department of Medicine, The University of North Carolina at Chapel Hill, Chapel Hill, North Carolina

HENRY KRUM, MBBS, PhD, FRACP, FCSANZ, FESC
Department of Epidemiology and Preventive Medicine, Centre of Cardiovascular Research and Education (CCRE) in Therapeutics, Alfred Hospital, Monash University, Melbourne, Victoria, Australia

TESS E. LIN, PharmD
Postdoctoral Fellow in Clinical Research and Drug Development, Division of Pharmacotherapy and Experimental Therapeutics, UNC Eshelman School of Pharmacy, The University of North Carolina (UNC) at Chapel Hill, Chapel Hill, North Carolina

ANTON LISHMANOV, MD, PhD
Division of Cardiology, Department of Medicine, The University of North Carolina at Chapel Hill, Chapel Hill, North Carolina

THOMAS J. O'NEILL, MD, PhD
Division of Cardiology, Department of Medicine, The University of North Carolina at Chapel Hill, Chapel Hill, North Carolina

KISHAN S. PARIKH, MD
Division of Cardiology, Duke University Medical Center, Durham, North Carolina

J. HERBERT PATTERSON, PharmD, FCCP
Professor of Pharmacy and Research Professor of Medicine; Executive Vice Chair, Division of Pharmacotherapy and Experimental Therapeutics, UNC Eshelman School of Pharmacy, The University of North Carolina (UNC) at Chapel Hill, Chapel Hill, North Carolina

PIERPAOLO PELLICORI, MD
Department of Cardiology, Hull York Medical School, Castle Hill Hospital, Kingston-upon-Hull, United Kingdom

BRENT N. REED, PharmD
Department of Pharmacy Practice and Science, University of Maryland School of Pharmacy, Baltimore, Maryland

JO E. RODGERS, PharmD
Division of Pharmacotherapy and Experimental Therapeutics, University of North Carolina Eshelman School of Pharmacy, Chapel Hill, North Carolina

JOHN J. ROMMEL, MD
Division of Cardiology, Department of Medicine, The University of North Carolina at Chapel Hill, Chapel Hill, North Carolina

LISA J. ROSE-JONES, MD
Assistant Professor, Advanced Heart Failure and Pulmonary Hypertension, UNC Heart and Vascular Center, Chapel Hill, North Carolina

SCOTT D. SOLOMON, MD
Cardiovascular Division, Brigham and Women's Hospital; Professor of Medicine, Harvard Medical School, Boston, Massachusetts

SARAH E. STREET, PhD
Department of Cell Biology and Physiology, University of North Carolina School of Medicine, Chapel Hill, North Carolina

CARLA A. SUETA, MD, PhD
UNC Center for Heart and Vascular Care, The University of North Carolina at Chapel Hill, Chapel Hill, North Carolina

ALI VAZIR, MB BS, PhD, MRCP
Cardiovascular Division, Brigham and Women's Hospital, Harvard Medical School, Boston, Massachusetts; NIHR Cardiovascular Biomedical Research Unit, Royal Brompton Hospital, Royal Brompton and Harefield NHS Foundation Trust, Institute of Cardiovascular Medicine and Sciences (ICMS), National Heart and Lung Institute (NHLI), Imperial College London, London, United Kingdom

Contents

The central roles of neurohormonal abnormalities in the pathobiology of heart failure have been defined in recent decades. Experiments have revealed both systemic involvement and intricate subcellular regulation by circulating effectors of the sympathetic nervous system, the renin-angiotensin-aldosterone system, and others. Randomized clinical trials substantiated these findings, establishing neurohormonal antagonists as cornerstones of heart failure pharmacotherapy, and occasionally offering further insight on mode of benefit. This review discusses the use of β-blockers, angiotensin-converting enzyme inhibitors, angiotensin receptor blockers, and aldosterone receptor antagonists in the treatment of heart failure, with particular attention to the pathophysiologic basis and mechanisms of action.

Mineralocorticoid receptor antagonists (MRAs) have become mandated therapy in patients with reduced ejection fraction (systolic) heart failure (HF) across all symptom classes. These agents should also be prescribed in the early post-myocardial infarction setting in those with reduced ejection fraction and either HF symptoms or diabetes. This article explores the pathophysiological role of aldosterone, an endogenous ligand for the mineralocorticoid receptor (MR), and summarizes the clinical data supporting guideline recommendations for these agents in systolic HF. The use of MRAs in novel areas beyond systolic HF ejection is also explored. Finally, the current status of newer agents will be examined.

The origins of the hydralazine/isosorbide dinitrate (H+ISDN) combination therapy are rooted in the first large-scale clinical trial in heart failure: V-HeFT I. Initially utilized for the balanced vasodilatory properties of each drug, we now know there is "more to the story." In fact, the maintenance of the nitroso-redox balance may be the true mechanism of benefit. Since the publication of V-HeFT I 30 years ago, H+ISDN has been the subject of much discussion and debate. Regardless of the many controversies surrounding H+ISDN, one thing is clear: therapy is underutilized and many patients who could benefit never receive the drugs. Ongoing physician and patient education are mandatory to improve the rates of H+ISDN use.

Polypharmacy, the use of 4 or more medications, is universal in patients with heart failure (HF). Evidence-based combination therapy is prescribed in patients with HF with reduced ejection fraction (HFrEF). Additionally, treatment of the high prevalence of comorbidities presents many therapeutic dilemmas. The use of nonprescription medications is common, adding further complexity to the medication therapy regimens of patients with HF. An approach for combining evidence-based therapies in patients with HFrEF is presented. Strategies for optimizing the management of common comorbidities in patients with HF are reviewed. Both prescription and nonprescription medications to avoid or use with caution are highlighted.

The management of heart failure with preserved ejection fraction (HFpEF) is challenging and requires an accurate diagnosis. Although currently there is no convincing therapy that prolongs survival in patients with HFpEF, treatment of fluid retention and of comorbidities, such as hypertension, myocardial ischemia, and atrial fibrillation, may improve symptoms and quality of life. Future outcome trials testing the efficacy of promising new agents will have better characterization of patient phenotype to maximize the potential response to therapies. This article provides current management strategies available for HFpEF, gives an overview of previous trials that have failed to prove the benefit of therapies to improve outcomes, and highlights promising novel therapies.

Pharmacogenomics explores one drug's varying effects on different patient genotypes. A better understanding of genomic variation's contribution to drug response can impact 4 arenas in heart failure (HF): (1) identification of patients most likely to receive benefit from therapy, (2) risk stratify patients for risk of adverse events, (3) optimize dosing of drugs, and (4) steer future clinical trial design and drug development. In this review, the authors explore the potential applications of pharmacogenomics in patients with HF in the context of these categories.

Hyponatremia is a known complication in patients with heart failure (HF). HF patients with severe congestion, hyponatremia, and renal insufficiency are difficult to manage and may have worse outcomes. A main cause of hyponatremia is inappropriately elevated level of plasma arginine vasopressin (AVP), which causes water retention at the collecting duct. AVP antagonists have thus been developed to increase aquaresis and serum sodium levels in patients with euvolemic and hypervolemic hyponatremia. Although tolvaptan, an AVP-2 receptor antagonist, did not show outcomes benefit in patients with decompensated HF, prospective studies are ongoing to evaluate its optimal role in targeted HF patients.

Interventions for coronary artery disease in heart failure have not been successful. It seems unlikely that coronary events play no role in the progression of heart failure and the ultimate demise of the patient. Meta-analysis suggests no benefit of fibrates in cardiovascular disease or heart failure. Polyunsaturated fats have equal benefit in cardiovascular disease. Two large trials of statins found no effect on mortality, but one trial found a reduction in morbidity. Retrospective analyses suggest that patients with milder disease might retain the benefit observed with statins in patients with coronary disease who do not have heart failure. Differences among statins may exist.

Atrial fibrillation (AF) is exceedingly common in patients with heart failure (HF), as they share common risk factors. Rate control is the cornerstone of treatment for AF; however, restoration of sinus rhythm should be considered when more than minimal symptoms are present. Life-threatening ventricular arrhythmias are responsible for the primary mode of death in patients with NYHA I, II, or III HF. Although implantable cardioverter defibrillators protect against sudden cardiac arrest, many patients will present with VT or ICD shocks. Antiarrhythmic drug therapy beyond beta-blocker therapy remains fundamental to the termination of acute VT and the prevention of ICD shocks.

Left ventricular assist devices (LVADs) are an increasingly common treatment for end-stage systolic heart failure. However, there are limited data on how to best treat patients pharmacologically after LVAD implantation, resulting in uncertainty about which heart failure medications provide the most benefit. Still, some evidence exists that certain medical therapies can prevent remodeling and improve right ventricular and, possibly, left ventricular function. This article reviews the current literature for medical heart failure therapy in LVAD patients, and possible future treatment strategies.

HEART FAILURE CLINICS

Foreword
Pharmacotherapy for Heart Failure: The More We Get to Know, the More We Need to Know

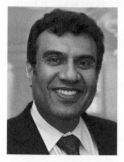
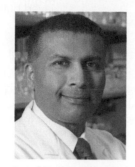

Mandeep R. Mehra, MD   Javed Butler, MD, MPH

Consulting Editors

To know, is to know that you know nothing.
That is the meaning of true knowledge.
—Socrates

It was not long ago, even in the early 1980s, that the treatment for patients with heart failure was largely restricted to the use of diuretics and digoxin. The past 3 decades have seen phenomenal progress in our understanding of heart failure pathophysiology, ranging across the spectrum of cardiac structural and functional abnormalities, neurohormonal activation, and systemic hemodynamic changes, to the effects of comorbidities on the progression of heart failure. These insights have led to targeted discoveries of novel therapies that have altered the entire natural history for patients suffering from heart failure.

As exhilarating as this rapid progress has been, scientific progress has raised many new poignant questions as well. Thus, ironically despite this progress, we have more questions about the management of heart failure patients than we did a couple of decades ago. Or perhaps this is due to the progress itself! These questions include the nature of interaction between emerging therapies,

their importance in subpopulations of heart failure patients, issues related to more personalized medicine, the impact of technology to discern the "omics" of heart failure patients, and obviously, the still unconquered frontier in heart failure with preserved ejection fraction.

In this issue of *Heart Failure Clinics* titled, "Pharmacologic Approaches to Heart Failure," Dr Kirkwood Adams has assembled highly experienced investigators and authors to address ten such discrete issues where, despite recent progress, several questions remained unanswered. This necessitated not only summarizing the existing data but also carefully extracting the themes and knowledge from these data, and their unique interpretation in light of the authors' experience. These topics include articles on existing therapies that are widely accepted, therapies that remain controversial, subpopulations for whom no known therapies exist, future direction in the "omics" era, and management challenges in patients taking multiple medications.

We are certain that this issue of *Heart Failure Clinics* will be an invaluable source for the readership in terms of improving care of the patients with

Heart Failure Clin 10 (2014) ix–x
http://dx.doi.org/10.1016/j.hfc.2014.07.011
1551-7136/14/$ – see front matter © 2014 Elsevier Inc. All rights reserved.

heart failure as well as a guide for future research in this field.

Mandeep R. Mehra, MD
Harvard Medical School
BWH Heart and Vascular Center
Center for Advanced Heart Disease
Brigham and Women's Hospital
75 Francis Street, A Building
3rd Floor, Room AB324
Boston, MA 02115, USA

Javed Butler, MD, MPH
Heart Failure Research
Emory Clinical Cardiovascular Research
Institute
Emory University
1462 Clifton Road NE, Suite 504
Atlanta, GA 30322, USA

E-mail addresses:
MMEHRA@partners.org (M.R. Mehra)
javed.butler@emory.edu (J. Butler)

Time and Technology Will Tell
The Pathophysiologic Basis of Neurohormonal Modulation in Heart Failure

Brent N. Reed, PharmD[a,1], Sarah E. Street, PhD[b,1],
Brian C. Jensen, MD[c,*]

KEYWORDS

- Heart failure • Sympathetic nervous system • Renin-angiotensin system • Drug therapy
- Physiology • Neurotransmitter agents • Adrenergic beta-antagonists
- Angiotensin-converting enzyme inhibitors

KEY POINTS

- Neurohormonal abnormalities are central to the pathobiology of heart failure and antagonism of their systemic effects is the basis of contemporary heart failure pharmacotherapy.
- β-Blockers likely confer benefit through induction of reverse remodeling, reduction of sudden cardiac death, and restoration of adaptive adrenergic signaling.
- Antagonists of the renin-angiotensin-aldosterone system have beneficial activities in cells of the heart in addition to their effects in the kidneys and peripheral vasculature.
- All agents that improve survival in heart failure target neurohormones, but not all neurohormonal modulators improve survival.

Healers have been treating heart failure (HF) for millennia, but the central role of neurohormonal abnormalities in its pathogenesis and management was discovered only recently.[1] HF previously was understood almost entirely as the result of structural and functional abnormalities of the heart. In the eighteenth century, anatomists described gross enlargement of failing hearts removed at autopsy, and concluded rightly that hypertrophy was central to the pathobiology of HF. Technological advances in the early twentieth century permitted evaluation of the beating heart, and the field of cardiac physiology evolved. As a result, HF came to be conceived in mechanical terms: the fundamental insult in the failing heart was impaired contractility, and this abnormality was either exacerbated or alleviated by alterations in load. Structure and function reconciled well in animal physiology laboratories, because the hypertrophied and failing heart both resulted from and led to altered loading conditions.

The essential role of neurohormonal disturbances in human HF was recognized first in the 1970s and brought to prominence in the 1980s and 1990s.[2] In this conception of HF, circulating substances synthesized in the heart, kidneys, adrenal glands, and pituitary glands engendered the characteristic anatomic and physiologic abnormalities described by earlier researchers. HF was no longer simply a disease of the heart.

Disclosure: The authors have no relevant financial disclosures.

[a] Department of Pharmacy Practice and Science, University of Maryland School of Pharmacy, 20 North Pine Street, Baltimore, MD 21201, USA; [b] Department of Cell Biology and Physiology, University of North Carolina School of Medicine, Chapel Hill, NC, USA; [c] Division of Cardiology and McAllister Heart Institute, University of North Carolina School of Medicine, 160 Dental Circle, Chapel Hill, NC 27599-7075, USA

[1] These authors contributed equally.

* Corresponding author.

E-mail address: bcjensen@med.unc.edu

Heart Failure Clin 10 (2014) 543–557
http://dx.doi.org/10.1016/j.hfc.2014.07.002

Increased levels of aldosterone and vasopressin explained the chronically increased preload in the failing heart; norepinephrine and angiotensin (Ang) II induced pathologic hypertrophy and detrimental increases in afterload.

Randomized clinical trials (another important technological advance) reinforced the neurohormonal paradigm. In 1987, the CONSENSUS (Cooperative North Scandinavian Enalapril Survival Study) showed a 31% reduction in 1-year mortality in patients with end-stage HF treated with the angiotensin-converting enzyme (ACE) inhibitor, enalapril, confirming the importance of Ang II in the progression of HF.[3] The use of beta-adrenergic receptor blockers (β-blockers) in HF was described first in 1981,[4] although the first large mortality trial of β-blockers in HF was the MDC (Metoprolol in Dilated Cardiomyopathy) trial, published in 1993.[5] MDC was followed in the next decade by the MERIT-HF (Metoprolol CR/XL Randomized Intervention Trial in Congestive Heart Failure), the US Carvedilol HF trials, CIBIS (Cardiac Insufficiency Bisoprolol Study) I and II, and COPERNICUS (Carvedilol Prospective Randomized Cumulative Survival) trial, collectively proving that β-blockers improve survival in HF (reviewed in Ref.[6]).

In many respects, clinical trial data have provided the strongest endorsement of the neurohormonal paradigm. Drugs that alter hemodynamic parameters without blocking neurohormonal activation, including digoxin,[7] non–potassium-sparing diuretics,[8] and positive inotropes,[9] have either neutral or negative effects on survival. In this respect, the contemporary use of neurohormonal modulators for HF pharmacotherapy offers an excellent example of reciprocity in translational science: elucidation of basic pathophysiology directs therapeutic targeting, and clinical trial results further inform the understanding of drug mechanism. This article discusses mechanisms of action for neurohormonal antagonists, with attention to both fundamental physiology and clinical trial outcomes.

THE SYMPATHETIC NERVOUS SYSTEM AND CARDIOVASCULAR PHYSIOLOGY

The sympathetic nervous system (SNS) is activated via arterial and venous baroreceptors and arterial chemoreceptors in response to decreases in perfusion pressure or oxygen delivery. In response, efferent fibers increase the release of norepinephrine (NE) (80%) or epinephrine (EPI) (20%) from synaptic varicosities in the myocardium and blood vessels, and stimulate the adrenal medulla to release NE (20%) and EPI (80%) into the blood. These hormones bind at least 9 different subtypes

of adrenergic receptors (ARs) (3 beta-ARs [β1, β2, β3], 3 alpha-1 ARs [α1A, α1B, α1D], and 3 alpha-2 ARs [α2A, α2B, α2C]) that are expressed variably by most cell types in the cardiovascular system and function primarily through G protein–coupled signaling cascades (**Fig. 1**).[10]

β1-ARs predominate in the myocardium (70%–80% of total β-ARs), whereas β2-ARs and β3-ARs are less abundant (15%–18% and 2%–3% respectively) (see **Fig. 1A**).[11] The predominant β-AR in vascular tissue is β2-AR, which mediates vasorelaxation (see **Fig. 1B**). Stimulation of β1-ARs on cardiomyocytes activates stimulatory G protein (Gs) and protein kinase A (PKA), leading to increased contractility (via activation of L-type calcium channels and ryanodine receptors); heart rate (via stimulation of L-type calcium channels and hyperpolarization-activated cyclic nucleotide-gated [HCN] channels); and rate of relaxation (via indirect stimulation of sarcoplasmic/endoplasmic reticulum calcium ATPase [SERCA] and Na/K-ATPase). Cardiomyocyte β2-AR activation also increases inotropy, although these receptors are less abundant and have a lower affinity for NE. The β2 is the predominant AR on cardiac fibroblasts, in which it likely plays important roles in HF pathobiology. β3-ARs exert an exclusively negative inotropic effect through activation of nitric oxide.[12]

α1-ARs are best known for their effects in vascular smooth muscle, where they promote vasoconstriction through activation of Gq, although myocardial α1-ARs mediate broadly beneficial effects, including positive inotropy, physiologic cardiomyocyte hypertrophy, and protection from cell death.[13] α2-ARs are predominantly found in presynaptic terminals of adrenergic neurons and adrenal chromaffin cells, where they inhibit NE/EPI release via Gi-related signaling cascades that inhibit PKA activation.[11,14] In this respect, α2-ARs negatively regulate excess NE/EPI release and spillover in both central and peripheral adrenergic synapses.

THE SNS AND HF PATHOPHYSIOLOGY

Chronic catecholamine excess is central to the pathobiology of HF, and the degree of activation is directly proportional to disease severity.[15,16] SNS upregulation also extends to the central nervous system, where NE spillover and turnover is increased.[17,18] In the periphery, SNS upregulation is organ specific: it is preferentially activated in cardiac tissue in mild to moderate HF, and only becomes activated in the kidney and other organ systems in severe HF.[19,20]

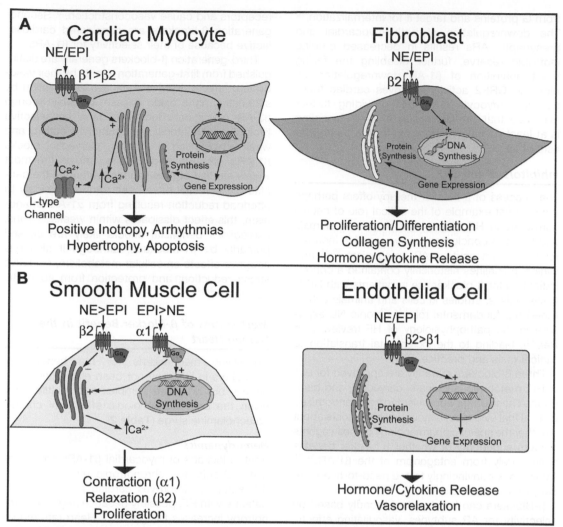

Fig. 1. SNS effector hormones and adrenergic receptor subtypes in cells of the (A) heart and (B) peripheral vasculature.

Chronic activation of cardiac β-ARs leads to pathologic cardiac hypertrophy and fibrosis: the hallmarks of ventricular remodeling. Increased levels of both local and circulating catecholamines lead to cardiac hypertrophy by acting directly on the cardiomyocyte β1-ARs[21] or by stimulating the paracrine release of other hormones such as Ang II and endothelin-1 (ET-1).[22] SNS activation also leads to direct stimulation of β2-ARs on cardiac fibroblasts, leading to fibroblast proliferation and increased release of cytokines such as interleukin-6, and hormones such as Ang II and ET-1. These factors in turn lead to increased collagen deposition, fibrosis, pathologic differentiation of fibroblasts into myofibroblasts, and cardiomyocyte hypertrophy.[23] Furthermore, chronic β1-AR hyperstimulation in animal models leads to necrotic and apoptotic cardiomyocyte death,

implicating sustained SNS activity in another important cellular mechanism of HF.[24]

Upregulation of the SNS can also cause ventricular arrhythmias[25] via direct effects on cardiomyocyte calcium handling mediated in part by catecholamine-induced ryanodine receptor dysfunction.[26] Chronic catecholamine surge can also promote both atrial and ventricular arrhythmias in HF indirectly through increased fibrosis and remodeling.[27]

Chronic myocardial β1-AR activation ultimately results in the depletion of NE from cardiac nerve terminals, and downregulation of myocardial β-ARs.[28] The desensitization and inactivation of membrane-bound β-ARs is performed by G protein–coupled receptor kinases (GRKs) that phosphorylate ARs, facilitating binding to beta-arrestins that uncouple the receptor from G proteins and target it for internalization.[10] The downregulation of both myocardial and presynaptic ARs results in decreased cardiac inotropic reserve, further disabling the failing heart. Inhibition of β1-AR downregulation by blocking GRK2 activity improves cardiac function and myocyte survival,[29] providing further evidence that the diminution of β-AR signaling is at least partially responsible for the pathogenesis of HF.

Inhibitors of the SNS

The success of β-blocker therapy offers perhaps the clearest example of the critical role of neurohormones in HF. Physiologic studies in animals and humans conclusively show negative inotropy resulting from acute β-AR antagonism,[30,31] and clinical guidelines historically contained a contraindication for β-blocker use in patients with HF.[32] Nevertheless, studies in cells and animals established the fundamental role of chronic NE exposure in the pathophysiology of HF (reviewed in Ref.[33]), leading to the incremental translation to clinical trials and practice.

Three β-blockers currently are approved for use in HF: metoprolol succinate, carvedilol, and bisoprolol. These drugs were selected from randomized clinical trial evidence, although debate exists about whether the specific pharmacology of these agents confers superiority or whether β-blocker benefits arise purely from antagonism of the β1-AR.[34,35] No trial has convincingly tested head-to-head efficacy of multiple β-blockers in HF.[36]

β-Blockers can be classified broadly based on selectivity for AR subtypes, vasodilating effects, and intrinsic sympathomimetic or sympatholytic properties (**Table 1**). First-generation β-blockers are not as well-tolerated in patients with HF, possibly as a result of blockade of vascular β2 receptors, which may shunt catecholamines to α1

receptors and cause vasoconstriction.[37] Second-generation β-blockers are considered cardioselective because of their selectivity for β1-ARs.

Third-generation β-blockers generally are distinguished from first-generation agents by their vasodilating effects. Nebivolol causes vasodilation by stimulating nitric oxide release, possibly through β3-AR activation. Bucindolol is a nonselective β-blocker with intrinsic sympatholytic activity and weak α1-blocking properties. Carvedilol blocks β1-ARs, β2-ARs, and α1-ARs, and is the most widely studied of these agents. Although the benefits of carvedilol have been attributed widely to afterload reduction resulting from α1-AR antagonism, this effect dissipates within weeks.[41] Thus, carvedilol's beneficial effects likely are caused primarily by β1-blockade, although it also has adaptive effects on cellular metabolism, oxidative stress reduction, and protection from apoptotic cell death.[45,46]

Mechanisms of β-Blocker Benefit in the Human Heart

Underlying mechanisms for the benefits of β-blockers in HF have not been elucidated completely, but likely are complex and multifactorial given the broadly pathologic effects of chronic catecholamine surge (**Table 2**).

Hemodynamics

Acute blockade of myocardial β1-ARs has negative inotropic and chronotropic effects. Chronic β-blocker use improves cardiac performance in patients with HF, possibly because negative chronotropy increases filling time.[66] Heart rate reduction has been used as an index of β-blocker efficacy and a meta-analysis of 23 randomized clinical trials indicates that heart rate reduction is a more powerful predictor of benefit than β-blocker dose. For every heart rate decrease of 5

Table 1
Classification and effects of β-blockers used in HF clinical trials

β-Blocker	β1 Block	β2 Block	α1 Block	Vascular Effects	Survival Benefit
First Generation					
Propranolol	+	+	−	None or vasoconstriction[37]	No
Second Generation					
Bisoprolol	+	−	−	None	Yes[38]
Metoprolol	+	−	−	None	Yes[39]
Third Generation					
Carvedilol	+	+	+	Acute: vasodilation[40] Chronic: none[41]	Yes[42]
Nebivolol	+	−	−	Vasodilation	No[43]
Bucindolol	+	+	+ (weak)	Vasodilation	No[44]

Table 2
Beneficial effects of neurohormonal antagonists in clinical trials of HF pharmacotherapy

Drug Class	Hemodynamic Effects	Remodeling Effects	Vascular Effects	Antiarrhythmic Effects
β-Blocker	↑EF[25,34] ↓Heart rate[47]	↓Volume[48–51]	Minimal	↓Arrhythmias ↓SCD[52] ↓ICD shocks[53,54]
ACE inhibitor or ARB	↑EF[55] ↓Afterload[56] ↓Preload[56]	↓Volume[55,57] ↓Hypertrophy[58]	↓Atheroma[59] ↓ACS[60] ↑Compliance	None
Aldosterone receptor antagonist	↑EF	± Volume[61] ↓Fibrosis[62,63]	↑Endothelial function	↓Arrhythmias[64,65] ↓SCD[64,65]

Abbreviations: ACS, acute coronary syndrome; ARB, angiotensin receptor blocker; EF, ejection fraction; ICD, implantable cardioverter defibrillator; SCD, sudden cardiac death.

beats per minute in the pooled β-blocker groups there was an 18% reduction in risk of death.[47] The early success of the specific HCN channel blocker ivabradine,[67] which slows heart rate without modulating the SNS, may corroborate the primary importance of negative chronotropy in HF therapy.

Chronic β-blocker use does not decrease contractile function in patients with HF. Invasive hemodynamic studies show improved stroke volume and cardiac index, at rest and peak exercise, after chronic carvedilol treatment.[68] A meta-analysis of 21 randomized clinical trials found an absolute increase in ejection fraction of 4% in patients with HF treated with β-blocker relative to placebo,[34] and a separate analysis of 18 trials reported a 29% relative increase in ejection fraction.[25] Ex vivo experiments on failing human heart tissue suggest that β-blocker use improves inotropic response to β-AR agonists and restores aspects of physiologic cardiomyocyte calcium handling[69] and responsiveness.[70] β-Blockers also improve the diastolic performance of the hypertrophied human heart.[71]

Reverse remodeling

Numerous clinical trials show the favorable effect of chronic β-blocker use on ventricular remodeling. In a MERIT-HF substudy, left ventricular (LV) end-diastolic volume index decreased by 17% and LV mass index decreased by almost 10% after 6 months of metoprolol.[48] Metoprolol also decreased LV end-diastolic index by 10% to 15% in patients with asymptomatic LV dysfunction in the REVERT (Reversal of Ventricular Remodeling with Toprol-XL) study.[49] Both CAPRICORN[50] and the Australia–New Zealand HF Research Collaborative Group[51] showed similar improvements with carvedilol.

β-Blockers decrease fibrosis in animal models of HF[72,73] and reduce circulating markers of fibrosis in humans,[74] although direct effects are not readily demonstrable in human hearts, perhaps because the β2-AR is the predominant AR on cardiac fibroblasts.

Antiarrhythmic effects

Sudden cardiac death is the primary cause of mortality in patients with New York Heart Association class I - III HF, and the well-established antiarrhythmic effects of β-blockers also contribute to their survival benefit. Although sudden cardiac death was not reduced in all trials of β-blockade in HF, a reduction was seen in the BHAT (Beta-Blocker Heart Attack Trial),[75] CAPRICORN,[76] CIBIS II,[38] and MERIT-HF.[39] A recent meta-analysis of 30 trials (24,779 patients) of β-blockers in HF found a 31% reduction in the risk of sudden cardiac death (odds ratio, 0.69; 95% confidence interval, 0.62–0.77) with a number needed to treat of 43 patients to prevent 1 sudden cardiac death per year.[52] β-Blocker use also substantially decreases the risk of both appropriate[53] and inappropriate defibrillator therapies.[54]

Molecular changes in human heart

Chronic β-blocker use in HF mitigates the characteristic decrease in myocardial β-AR abundance, although it is unclear whether this effect is essential for clinical or physiologic benefit.[66,77] β-Blocker use also abrogates the pathologic changes in gene expression in the failing heart: α-myosin heavy chain abundance increases, β-myosin heavy chain decreases, and sarcoplasmic reticulum Ca^{2+} ATPase levels are restored.[77]

Digoxin and the SNS

In the past, the usefulness of digoxin in HF has been attributed to its positive inotropic effects. However, these effects are only present at high serum digoxin concentrations (>1 ng/mL), at which an increased risk of mortality has also been observed.[78] It has been proposed that the benefits of digoxin at lower concentrations result in part from neurohormonal modulation. Among its many pharmacologic actions, digoxin decreases circulating norepinephrine and renin levels[79,80] and has a favorable impact on natriuretic peptide release.[81]

Risks of sympatholysis in HF

Although the essential role of catecholamine excess in the pathophysiology of HF is beyond dispute, direct sympatholytic therapies have been associated with poorer outcomes. In a study of patients with chronic HF, a sustained-release preparation of moxonidine, an imidazoline receptor agonist that reduces sympathetic outflow, improved ventricular performance but led to an increase in serious adverse events.[82] These risks were confirmed in a larger trial, which was terminated early because of a nearly 2-fold increase in death among those randomized to moxonidine.[83] The intrinsic sympatholytic properties of bucindolol may help explain why outcomes in the BEST (Beta-Blocker Evaluation in Survival Trial) were less favorable than those of other β-blocker clinical trials.[44]

One conceivable explanation for the apparent risk associated with sympatholysis is the abrogation of adaptive effects of myocardial α1-AR activation. Evidence from human studies suggests that the relative increase in α1-AR expression observed in advanced HF may be a compensatory response to preserve myocardial function in the setting of β1-AR downregulation and dysfunction.[84] These cardioprotective effects may explain why therapies that inhibit α1-ARs have been linked to adverse outcomes in patients with HF. An arm of ALLHAT that randomized patients to the α1-blocker doxazosin was stopped early for a 2-fold increase in incident HF.[85]

THE RENIN-ANGIOTENSIN-ALDOSTERONE SYSTEM AND CARDIOVASCULAR PHYSIOLOGY

The renin-angiotensin-aldosterone system (RAAS) consists of a protease cascade that is activated by renin release from the juxtaglomerular cells of renal afferent arterioles. Renin is secreted in response to decreased renal perfusion pressure, decreased salt delivery to the distal convoluted tubule, increased renal sympathetic nerve activity, or changes in circulating natriuretic peptides. Renin catalyzes the cleavage of angiotensinogen, a circulating protein produced by the liver. The

resulting peptide, angiotensin I (Ang I), is then cleaved by ACE, to generate Ang II, which is among the most potent endogenous vasoconstrictors. Ang II binds to 2 G protein–coupled receptors, angiotensin II receptor, type I (AT1) and AT2. AT1 is the primary receptor expressed on vascular smooth muscle, endothelium, myocardium, neurons, and fibroblasts, whereas AT2 is primarily expressed early in development and its effects are less well understood in adults.[86,87]

The other potent effector hormone of RAAS, aldosterone, is a steroid hormone released primarily from the adrenal cortex in response to increased Ang II and plasma [K+]. Aldosterone binds to the intracellular mineralocorticoid receptor (MR) leading to increased salt and water reabsorption, increased blood volume, and alterations in ion-channel expression.[88]

In the past, RAAS-associated hormones were considered to be renally controlled endocrine hormones that exerted effects widely throughout the body. However, it is now well understood that tissues such as the heart, blood vessels, lungs, and brain have an intrinsic RAAS that functions in an autocrine/paracrine manner.[89] In the heart, local stress, cellular damage, and stretch can each lead to an upregulation of locally produced RAAS components including ACE, Ang II, and aldosterone.[90,91] It is now thought that cardiac-generated RAAS components play a major role in the progression of HF.[92]

THE RAAS AND HF PATHOPHYSIOLOGY

Circulating and intrinsic Ang II and aldosterone are increased in HF, and contribute to HF pathophysiology through both extracardiac and direct cardiac effects.[92,93] In vascular tissue, Ang II and aldosterone mediate increased vasoconstriction, unfavorable vascular remodeling, and endothelial dysfunction (Fig. 2B).[94,95] Ang II and aldosterone promote sodium and water reabsorption in the proximal and distal convoluted tubules respectively. RAAS hormones also have important direct effects on myocardial cells.[96] Ang II induces cardiomyocyte hypertrophy and cardiac fibroblast proliferation through activation of AT1 receptors,[97] promoting cardiac hypertrophy independent of effects on blood pressure.[98] Aldosterone also promotes cardiac fibrosis through activation of mineralocorticoid receptors on cardiac fibroblasts (see Fig. 2A).

In addition to the directly deleterious effects of Ang II and aldosterone, RAAS also interacts with other neurohormonal signals that contribute to the pathobiology of HF. For example, local Ang II production leads to increased NE release from

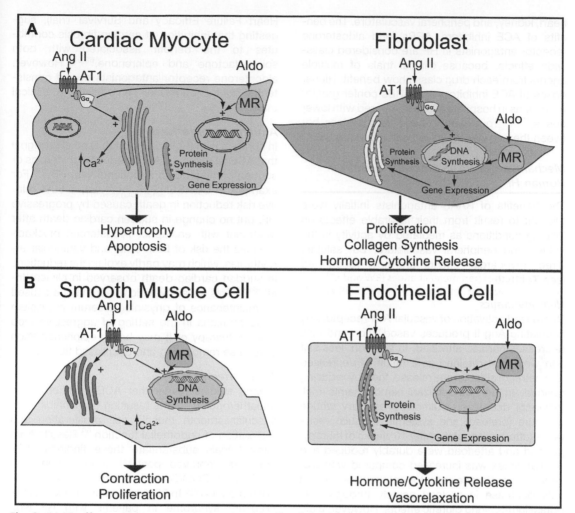

Fig. 2. RAAS effector hormones and receptors in cells of the (*A*) heart and (*B*) peripheral vasculature. Aldo, aldosterone.

sympathetic nerve terminals in the heart.[99] Ang II also has effects on the central nervous system, causing a central activation of sympathetic nerves that target the cardiovascular system.[100] Central inhibition of AT1 receptors leads to a decrease in sympathetic nerve activity in the heart.[101]

In addition to these well-known RAAS constituents, several other RAAS enzymes contribute to cardiovascular regulation. ACE2, neprilysin (also known as neutral endopeptidase),[87] prolylendopeptidases, and prolylcarboxypeptidases break down Ang I and II, ultimately leading to the generation of a peptide known as Ang(1–7).[87] Ang(1–7) acts on its own receptor, MasR, counteracting the effects of Ang II by causing vasodilation, decreased fibrosis, decreased oxidative stress, and decreased hypertrophy.[102] In addition to cleaving Ang I, ACE also is the main enzyme that breaks down the vasodilator bradykinin. It has

been proposed that one of the key mechanisms of ACE inhibitors in the treatment of HF is increasing bradykinin levels, directly leading to vasodilation and decreased afterload.[103] However, increased bradykinin is also responsible for several of the side effects of ACE inhibitor treatment such as angioedema and dry cough.[104]

Inhibitors of the RAAS

Inhibitors of RAAS used in the management of HF include ACE inhibitors, angiotensin receptor blockers (ARBs), and aldosterone receptor antagonists. ACE inhibitors prevent the conversion of Ang I to Ang II, whereas ARBs competitively inhibit the effect of Ang II on AT1 receptors in heart, kidney, and vascular tissue. Aldosterone receptor antagonists competitively inhibit the binding of aldosterone to mineralocorticoid receptors in the heart, kidney, and peripheral vasculature. The benefits of ACE inhibitors, ARBs, and aldosterone receptor antagonists in HF are considered class-wide effects, because clinical trials of multiple agents from each drug class show benefit. Higher doses of ACE inhibitors and ARBs confer greater reductions in hospitalizations compared with lower doses,[105,106] but head-to-head comparisons between the two classes have been inconclusive.

Mechanisms of RAAS Blockade Benefit in Human HF

The benefits of RAAS antagonists initially were thought to result from their favorable effects on loading conditions as mediated by activity in the kidney and peripheral vasculature, but salutary direct myocardial effects are now recognized (see **Table 2**).

Hemodynamics
Decreased activation of vascular AT1 receptors by circulating Ang II produces vasodilation and thus decreases cardiac afterload. In addition, less salt and water are retained as a result of decreased downstream aldosterone release, thereby reducing preload. In one randomized hemodynamic trial, fosinopril decreased pulmonary capillary wedge pressure (preload) and systemic vascular resistance (afterload) acutely. After 10 weeks of therapy, preload and afterload were durably reduced and cardiac index was increased compared with placebo.[56] Aldosterone receptor antagonists cause a mild decrease in preload acutely through their potassium-sparing diuretic effects. However, a clinically meaningful diuretic effect is less commonly observed at the low doses used in HF and is unlikely to explain the magnitude of benefit observed in clinical trials.

Reverse remodeling
ACE inhibitors and ARBs have uniformly favorable effects on cardiac remodeling in HF. In the SOLVD (Studies of Left Ventricular Dysfunction) trial, 1 year of enalapril resulted in a 10% decrease in both LV end-diastolic and end-systolic volumes.[57] Similar results were reported with post-MI treatment with captopril in SAVE (Survival and Ventricular Enlargement) trial.[107] Losartan led to greater regression of LV hypertrophy than atenolol in the LIFE (Losartan Intervention For Endpoint) trial,[58] and treatment with valsartan led to decreased ventricular volume and increased ejection fraction in Val-HeFT (Valsartan Heart Failure Trial).[55]

Aldosterone receptor antagonists reduced circulating markers of collagen turnover in both RALES (Randomized Aldactone Evaluation Study) and EPHESUS (Eplerenone Post-AMI

Heart Failure Efficacy and Survival Trial), suggesting that inhibition of cardiac fibrosis contributes to the benefit associated with both spironolactone and eplerenone.[62,63] However, aldosterone receptor antagonists do not consistently confer beneficial remodeling in clinical trials.[61]

Antiarrhythmic effects
In contrast with β-blockers, there is no clear signal that ACE inhibitors or ARBs reduce arrhythmias or sudden cardiac death in patients with HF.[108] For example, in CONSENSUS there was a 50% relative risk reduction in death caused by progressive HF, but no change in sudden cardiac death after treatment with enalapril.[3] Aldosterone blockade reduces the risk of both atrial and ventricular arrhythmias, which may partly explain the reductions in sudden cardiac death observed in clinical trials.[64,65] This antiarrhythmic effect may be caused by maintenance of physiologic serum potassium concentrations in the setting of aggressive loop diuretic therapy or it may be an epiphenomenon of reverse remodeling and decreased fibrosis.

Other effects
Animal studies reveal that ACE inhibitors have antiatherogenic effects resulting from inhibition of vascular smooth muscle cell proliferation and restoration of endothelial function.[59] Results from clinical trials substantiate these findings. ACE inhibitors improved post-MI outcomes in both SAVE and SOLVD and a large meta-analysis confirmed a 20% to 25% reduction in risk of acute coronary syndrome in patients with HF who received an ACE inhibitor.[60] ACE inhibitors also delay progression of renal dysfunction, which is a harbinger of poor outcome in HF.[109]

ACE (aldosterone) escape
The efficacy of RAAS antagonists can diminish over time through an effect known as aldosterone or ACE escape, whereby a maladaptive increase in RAAS components is observed after chronic treatment with RAAS antagonists.[110] ACE escape occurs in approximately 10% of patients within 6 months and 50% of patients within 12 months of starting treatment.[111] There are several potential physiologic explanations for this phenomenon. Prolonged inhibition of ACE or AT1 leads to increased levels of renin and Ang I because of the loss of negative feedback by Ang II. In the setting of ACE inhibition, several other enzymes such as chymase and cathepsin also cleave circulating and local Ang I to Ang II, leading to aldosterone production (escape).[104]

Further, a receptor for renin and prorenin (inactive renin) has recently been discovered. Binding of (pro)renin to the (pro)renin receptor (PRR) leads to increased fibrosis and release of cytokines and prohypertrophic growth factors. PRR also serves an enzymatic function, generating active renin from inactive (pro)renin.[112]

Multiple clinical trials have investigated the possibility that dual RAAS antagonist therapy could abrogate ACE escape and improve outcomes in HF. Combined treatment with ACE inhibitor and ARB produced incremental improvements in cardiovascular mortality and hospitalizations but was also associated with an increase in adverse events.[113,114] Meta-analysis of 4 published clinical trials of RAAS combination therapy found a 2-fold increased risk of worsening renal function and a nearly 5-fold higher risk of hyperkalemia,[115] likely caused by pronounced decreases in circulating aldosterone levels.

The compensatory increase in renin release in the setting of ACE inhibitor and/or ARB therapy has also prompted trials of direct renin inhibitors (DRIs) in patients with HF. It was postulated that renin inhibition would augment downstream RAAS blockade and provide additive benefits when combined with ACE inhibitor or ARB therapy. Although the DRI aliskiren reduces plasma renin activity, there is no evidence of a clinical benefit in HF. In ASTRONAUT (Aliskiren Trial on Acute Heart Failure Outcomes), a large randomized controlled clinical trial of patients on optimal HF therapy (including other RAAS antagonists), aliskiren failed to reduce a composite of cardiovascular death or hospitalizations and was associated with hypotension, renal dysfunction, and hyperkalemia.[116] ATMOSPHERE (Aliskiren Trial of Minimizing Outcomes for Patients with Heart Failure), a trial comparing aliskiren with enalapril in patients with HF is underway.[117]

NATRIURETIC PEPTIDES AND CARDIOVASCULAR PHYSIOLOGY

The natriuretic peptides (atrial natriuretic peptide [ANP], B-type natriuretic peptide [BNP], and C-type natriuretic peptide [CNP]) collectively produce adaptive effects in HF and oppose the actions of the effector hormones of the SNS and RAAS. ANP is released by cells in the atrial wall in response to stretch or increases in plasma Ang II, ET-1, and vasopressin.[118] BNP is released primarily from the left ventricle, although atrial cells also release BNP at a much lower concentration than ANP.[119] CNP is released by endothelial cells in response to increased cytokines and other hormones such as acetylcholine.[120] ANP, BNP, and CNP bind to 2 transmembrane-bound guanylyl cyclases (GCs), GC-A and GC-B, to increase

intracellular cyclic guanosine monophosphate (cGMP) and elicit wide-ranging physiologic effects including vasodilation, increased salt and water excretion, decreased renin release, dampened SNS activity, decreased cardiac fibrosis, and blunted cardiomyocyte hypertrophy.[121–125]

Targeting Natriuretic Peptides for HF Therapy

Nesiritide is a recombinant form of BNP that binds GC receptors on vascular endothelium and in the kidney. Nesiritide mimics the salutary effects of endogenous BNP on cardiovascular hemodynamics and renal physiology, but does not reduce symptoms to a significantly greater extent than diuretics and vasodilators.[126] In large clinical trials, nesiritide did not improve survival, although early concerns over increased mortality and worsening renal function have subsided.

BNP has a short plasma half-life because of its removal by cellular reuptake, the natriuretic peptide clearance receptor (GC-C), and breakdown by neprilysin, the same enzyme that generates Ang(1–7) from Ang I.[127] Neprilysin inhibitors have been developed in an attempt to increase the half-life of circulating BNP for therapeutic benefit, although they typically also have been designed to antagonize RAAS in order to counter the unfavorable effects of decreased Ang(1–7) levels. Omapatrilat, a vasopeptide inhibitor of both neprilysin and ACE, exerted favorable hemodynamic effects, but was associated with a more than 3-fold increase in angioedema compared with an ACE inhibitor, likely caused by its inhibition of both bradykinin and substance P degradation.[128] The focus has since shifted to compounds that both inhibit neprilysin and block Ang II receptors. A study comparing enalapril and LCZ696, a dual neprilysin inhibitor and ARB, in chronic HF is underway.[129]

VASOPRESSIN IN HF PATHOPHYSIOLOGY AND PHARMACOTHERAPY

Vasopressin (arginine vasopressin [AVP]) is released in response to increased osmolarity, Ang II, or SNS stimulation, and is chronically increased in HF.[130] AVP is secreted primarily from the posterior pituitary, but local vasopressin production may also contribute to the progression of HF.[131] Vasopressin stimulates the activity of 3 G protein–coupled receptors, $V1_a$, $V1_b$, and V2. $V1_a$, expressed on vascular smooth muscle and ventricular myocardium, couples to G_q, increasing intracellular calcium and causing vasoconstriction, positive inotropy, and hypertrophy.[132] The V2 receptor mediates free water reabsorption in the kidney. Excess stimulation can lead to hypervolemic hyponatremia in patients with HF.

Recognition that AVP secretion is upregulated in HF prompted investigations of vasopressin receptor antagonists (VRAs) as another novel therapeutic strategy. Despite aggressive diuretic therapy, many patients with HF continue to retain excess free water and hyponatremia is common. However, whether hyponatremia represents a target of pharmacologic therapy or a surrogate marker for the severity of disease remains an area of controversy. VRAs competitively inhibit V_2 receptors in renal collecting ducts, thereby preventing the reabsorption of free water. Tolvaptan, an oral VRA, is selective for V_2 receptors, whereas intravenous conivaptan also inhibits V_{1A} receptors. In EVEREST (Efficacy of Vasopressin Antagonism in Heart Failure Outcome Study with Tolvaptan), tolvaptan conferred improvements in some HF symptoms, but did not improve survival.[133] Although tolvaptan partially corrects hyponatremia, the effect is not durable after discontinuation of therapy.[134] The reasons for the modest clinical impact of this physiologically rational therapeutic approach are unclear.

SUMMARY

The depth to which disease mechanism is understood is often dictated by extant technologies. In that respect, the conception of HF was informed successively by gross anatomy, organ-level physiology, and cellular physiology. As outlined in this review, recent advances have enabled an expansion in knowledge of the cellular and subcellular mechanisms that underlie the characteristic neurohormonal disturbances in HF. How will today's emerging technologies influence understanding of HF? Will massively parallel sequencing technologies inform clinicians that HF fundamentally is a disease of genetic and epigenetic modifications?[135,136] Will the next generation of HF therapies target DNA methylation? Epigenetic reader proteins?[137] Noncoding RNAs or microRNAs?[138] As always, only time will tell.

REFERENCES

1. Katz AM. The "modern" view of heart failure: how did we get here? Circ Heart Fail 2008;1(1):63–71.
2. Francis GS, Goldsmith SR, Levine TB, et al. The neurohumoral axis in congestive heart failure. Ann Intern Med 1984;101(3):370–7.
3. Effects of enalapril on mortality in severe congestive heart failure. Results of the Cooperative North Scandinavian Enalapril Survival Study (CONSENSUS). The CONSENSUS Trial Study Group. N Engl J Med 1987;316(23):1429–35.
4. Ikram H, Fitzpatrick D. Double-blind trial of chronic oral beta blockade in congestive cardiomyopathy. Lancet 1981;2(8245):490–3.
5. Waagstein F, Bristow MR, Swedberg K, et al. Beneficial effects of metoprolol in idiopathic dilated cardiomyopathy. Metoprolol in Dilated Cardiomyopathy (MDC) Trial Study Group. Lancet 1993;342(8885):1441–6.
6. Foody JM, Farrell MH, Krumholz HM. beta-Blocker therapy in heart failure: scientific review. JAMA 2002;287(7):883–9.
7. Digitalis Investigation Group. The effect of digoxin on mortality and morbidity in patients with heart failure. N Engl J Med 1997;336(8):525–33.
8. Domanski M, Norman J, Pitt B, et al. Diuretic use, progressive heart failure, and death in patients in the Studies Of Left Ventricular Dysfunction (SOLVD). J Am Coll Cardiol 2003;42(4):705–8.
9. Felker GM, O'Connor CM. Inotropic therapy for heart failure: an evidence-based approach. Am Heart J 2001;142(3):393–401.
10. Lymperopoulos A, Rengo G, Koch WJ. Adrenergic nervous system in heart failure: pathophysiology and therapy. Circ Res 2013;113(6):739–53.
11. Rockman HA, Koch WJ, Lefkowitz RJ. Seven-transmembrane-spanning receptors and heart function. Nature 2002;415(6868):206–12.
12. Gauthier C, Leblais V, Kobzik L, et al. The negative inotropic effect of beta3-adrenoceptor stimulation is mediated by activation of a nitric oxide synthase pathway in human ventricle. J Clin Invest 1998; 102(7):1377–84.
13. Jensen BC, O'Connell TD, Simpson PC. Alpha-1-adrenergic receptors in heart failure: the adaptive arm of the cardiac response to chronic catecholamine stimulation. J Cardiovasc Pharmacol 2014; 63(4):291–301.
14. Lymperopoulos A, Rengo G, Koch WJ. Adrenal adrenoceptors in heart failure: fine-tuning cardiac stimulation. Trends Mol Med 2007;13(12):503–11.
15. Cohn JN, Levine TB, Olivari MT, et al. Plasma norepinephrine as a guide to prognosis in patients with chronic congestive heart failure. N Engl J Med 1984;311(13):819–23.
16. Kaye DM, Lefkovits J, Jennings GL, et al. Adverse consequences of high sympathetic nervous activity in the failing human heart. J Am Coll Cardiol 1995; 26(5):1257–63.
17. Kaye DM, Lambert GW, Lefkovits J, et al. Neurochemical evidence of cardiac sympathetic activation and increased central nervous system norepinephrine turnover in severe congestive heart failure. J Am Coll Cardiol 1994;23(3):570–8.
18. Aggarwal A, Esler MD, Lambert GW, et al. Norepinephrine turnover is increased in suprabulbar subcortical brain regions and is related to whole-body sympathetic activity in human heart failure. Circulation 2002;105(9):1031–3.

19. Ramchandra R, Hood SG, Denton DA, et al. Basis for the preferential activation of cardiac sympathetic nerve activity in heart failure. Proc Natl Acad Sci U S A 2009;106(3):924–8.

20. Rundqvist B, Elam M, Bergmann-Sverrisdottir Y, et al. Increased cardiac adrenergic drive precedes generalized sympathetic activation in human heart failure. Circulation 1997;95(1):169–75.

21. Ju H, Zhao S, Tappia PS, et al. Expression of Gq alpha and PLC-beta in scar and border tissue in heart failure due to myocardial infarction. Circulation 1998;97(9):892–9.

22. Sutton MG, Sharpe N. Left ventricular remodeling after myocardial infarction: pathophysiology and therapy. Circulation 2000;101(25):2981–8.

23. Porter KE, Turner NA. Cardiac fibroblasts: at the heart of myocardial remodeling. Pharmacol Ther 2009;123(2):255–78.

24. Singh K, Xiao L, Remondino A, et al. Adrenergic regulation of cardiac myocyte apoptosis. J Cell Physiol 2001;189(3):257–65.

25. Lechat P, Packer M, Chalon S, et al. Clinical effects of beta-adrenergic blockade in chronic heart failure: a meta-analysis of double-blind, placebo-controlled, randomized trials. Circulation 1998; 98(12):1184–91.

26. Blayney LM, Lai FA. Ryanodine receptor-mediated arrhythmias and sudden cardiac death. Pharmacol Ther 2009;123(2):151–77.

27. Jessup M, Brozena S. Heart failure. N Engl J Med 2003;348(20):2007–18.

28. Bristow MR, Ginsburg R, Minobe W, et al. Decreased catecholamine sensitivity and beta-adrenergic-receptor density in failing human hearts. N Engl J Med 1982;307(4):205–11.

29. Akhter SA, Eckhart AD, Rockman HA, et al. In vivo inhibition of elevated myocardial beta-adrenergic receptor kinase activity in hybrid transgenic mice restores normal beta-adrenergic signaling and function. Circulation 1999;100(6):648–53.

30. Epstein S, Robinson BF, Kahler RL, et al. Effects of beta-adrenergic blockade on the cardiac response to maximal and submaximal exercise in man. J Clin Invest 1965;44(11):1745–53.

31. Nayler WG, Chipperfield D, Lowe TE. The negative inotropic effect of adrenergic betareceptor blocking drugs on human heart muscle. Cardiovasc Res 1969;3(1):30–6.

32. Guidelines for the evaluation and management of heart failure. Report of the American College of Cardiology/American Heart Association Task Force on Practice Guidelines (Committee on Evaluation and Management of Heart Failure). Circulation 1995;92(9):2764–84.

33. Pool PE, Braunwald E. Fundamental mechanisms in congestive heart failure. Am J Cardiol 1968; 22(1):7–15.

34. Chatterjee S, Biondi-Zoccai G, Abbate A, et al. Benefits of beta blockers in patients with heart failure and reduced ejection fraction: network meta-analysis. BMJ 2013;346:f55.

35. Khazanie P, Newby LK. ACP Journal Club. Review: in patients with heart failure, beta-blockers reduce mortality but do not differ from each other. Ann Intern Med 2013;158(10):JC2–3.

36. Poole-Wilson PA, Swedberg K, Cleland JG, et al. Comparison of carvedilol and metoprolol on clinical outcomes in patients with chronic heart failure in the Carvedilol Or Metoprolol European Trial (COMET): randomised controlled trial. Lancet 2003;362(9377): 7–13.

37. Bristow MR. β-Adrenergic receptor blockade in chronic heart failure. Circulation 2000;101(5):558–69.

38. The Cardiac Insufficiency Bisoprolol Study II (CIBIS-II): a randomised trial. Lancet 1999;353(9146):9–13.

39. Effect of metoprolol CR/XL in chronic heart failure: Metoprolol CR/XL Randomised Intervention Trial in Congestive Heart Failure (MERIT-HF). Lancet 1999;353(9169):2001–7.

40. Yue TL, Cheng HY, Lysko PG, et al. Carvedilol, a new vasodilator and beta adrenoceptor antagonist, is an antioxidant and free radical scavenger. J Pharmacol Exp Ther 1992;263(1):92–8.

41. Kubo T, Azevedo ER, Newton GE, et al. Lack of evidence for peripheral alpha(1)-adrenoceptor blockade during long-term treatment of heart failure with carvedilol. J Am Coll Cardiol 2001;38(5): 1463–9.

42. Packer M, Bristow MR, Cohn JN, et al. The effect of carvedilol on morbidity and mortality in patients with chronic heart failure. U.S. Carvedilol Heart Failure Study Group. N Engl J Med 1996;334(21): 1349–55.

43. Flather MD, Shibata MC, Coats AJ, et al. Randomized trial to determine the effect of nebivolol on mortality and cardiovascular hospital admission in elderly patients with heart failure (SENIORS). Eur Heart J 2005;26(3):215–25.

44. Beta-Blocker Evaluation of Survival Trial Investigators. A trial of the beta-blocker bucindolol in patients with advanced chronic heart failure. N Engl J Med 2001;344(22):1659–67.

45. Nakamura K, Kusano K, Nakamura Y, et al. Carvedilol decreases elevated oxidative stress in human failing myocardium. Circulation 2002;105(24):2867–71.

46. Wang R, Miura T, Harada N, et al. Pleiotropic effects of the beta-adrenoceptor blocker carvedilol on calcium regulation during oxidative stress-induced apoptosis in cardiomyocytes. J Pharmacol Exp Ther 2006;318(1):45–52.

47. McAlister FA, Wiebe N, Ezekowitz JA, et al. Meta-analysis: beta-blocker dose, heart rate reduction, and death in patients with heart failure. Ann Intern Med 2009;150(11):784–94.

48. Groenning BA, Nilsson JC, Sondergaard L, et al. Antiremodeling effects on the left ventricle during beta-blockade with metoprolol in the treatment of chronic heart failure. J Am Coll Cardiol 2000; 36(7):2072–80.

49. Colucci WS, Kolias TJ, Adams KF, et al. Metoprolol reverses left ventricular remodeling in patients with asymptomatic systolic dysfunction: the REversal of VEntricular Remodeling with Toprol-XL (REVERT) trial. Circulation 2007;116(1):49–56.

50. Doughty RN, Whalley GA, Walsh HA, et al. Effects of carvedilol on left ventricular remodeling after acute myocardial infarction: the CAPRICORN Echo Substudy. Circulation 2004;109(2):201–6.

51. Doughty RN, Whalley GA, Gamble G, et al. Left ventricular remodeling with carvedilol in patients with congestive heart failure due to ischemic heart disease. Australia-New Zealand Heart Failure Research Collaborative Group. J Am Coll Cardiol 1997;29(5):1060–6.

52. Al-Gobari M, El Khatib C, Pillon F, et al. Beta-blockers for the prevention of sudden cardiac death in heart failure patients: a meta-analysis of randomized controlled trials. BMC Cardiovasc Disord 2013;13:52.

53. Friedman DJ, Altman RK, Orencole M, et al. Predictors of sustained ventricular arrhythmias in cardiac resynchronization therapy. Circ Arrhyth Electrophysiol 2012;5(4):762–72.

54. Ruwald MH, Abu-Zeitone A, Jons C, et al. Impact of carvedilol and metoprolol on inappropriate implantable cardioverter-defibrillator therapy: the MADIT-CRT trial (Multicenter Automatic Defibrillator Implantation with Cardiac Resynchronization Therapy). J Am Coll Cardiol 2013;62(15):1343–50.

55. Wong M, Staszewsky L, Latini R, et al. Valsartan benefits left ventricular structure and function in heart failure: Val-HeFT echocardiographic study. J Am Coll Cardiol 2002;40(5):970–5.

56. Sharma S, Deitchman D, Eni JS, et al. The hemodynamic effects of long-term ACE inhibition with fosinopril in patients with heart failure. Fosinopril Hemodynamics Study Group. Am J Ther 1999; 6(4):181–9.

57. Konstam MA, Rousseau MF, Kronenberg MW, et al. Effects of the angiotensin converting enzyme inhibitor enalapril on the long-term progression of left ventricular dysfunction in patients with heart failure. SOLVD Investigators. Circulation 1992;86(2):431–8.

58. Devereux RB, Dahlof B, Gerdts E, et al. Regression of hypertensive left ventricular hypertrophy by losartan compared with atenolol: the Losartan Intervention for Endpoint Reduction in Hypertension (LIFE) trial. Circulation 2004;110(11):1456–62.

59. Pitt B. Potential role of angiotensin converting enzyme inhibitors in treatment of atherosclerosis. Eur Heart J 1995;16(Suppl K):49–54.

60. Teo KK, Yusuf S, Pfeffer M, et al. Effects of long-term treatment with angiotensin-converting-enzyme inhibitors in the presence or absence of aspirin: a systematic review. Lancet 2002;360(9339):1037–43.

61. Udelson JE, Feldman AM, Greenberg B, et al. Randomized, double-blind, multicenter, placebo-controlled study evaluating the effect of aldosterone antagonism with eplerenone on ventricular remodeling in patients with mild-to-moderate heart failure and left ventricular systolic dysfunction. Circ Heart Fail 2010;3(3):347–53.

62. Zannad F, Alla F, Dousset B, et al. Limitation of excessive extracellular matrix turnover may contribute to survival benefit of spironolactone therapy in patients with congestive heart failure: insights from the Randomized Aldactone Evaluation Study (RALES). Rales Investigators. Circulation 2000;102(22):2700–6.

63. Iraqi W, Rossignol P, Angioi M, et al. Extracellular cardiac matrix biomarkers in patients with acute myocardial infarction complicated by left ventricular dysfunction and heart failure: insights from the Eplerenone Post-Acute Myocardial Infarction Heart Failure Efficacy and Survival Study (EPHESUS) study. Circulation 2009;119(18):2471–9.

64. Shah NC, Pringle SD, Donnan PT, et al. Spironolactone has antiarrhythmic activity in ischaemic cardiac patients without cardiac failure. J Hypertens 2007;25(11):2345–51.

65. Swedberg K, Zannad F, McMurray JJ, et al. Eplerenone and atrial fibrillation in mild systolic heart failure: results from the EMPHASIS-HF (Eplerenone in Mild Patients Hospitalization And SurvIval Study in Heart Failure) study. J Am Coll Cardiol 2012;59(18): 1598–603.

66. Gilbert EM, Abraham WT, Olsen S, et al. Comparative hemodynamic, left ventricular functional, and antiadrenergic effects of chronic treatment with metoprolol versus carvedilol in the failing heart. Circulation 1996;94(11):2817–25.

67. Fox K, Komajda M, Ford I, et al. Effect of ivabradine in patients with left-ventricular systolic dysfunction: a pooled analysis of individual patient data from the BEAUTIFUL and SHIFT trials. Eur Heart J 2013;34(29):2263–70.

68. Metra M, Nardi M, Giubbini R, et al. Effects of short- and long-term carvedilol administration on rest and exercise hemodynamic variables, exercise capacity and clinical conditions in patients with idiopathic dilated cardiomyopathy. J Am Coll Cardiol 1994; 24(7):1678–87.

69. Reiken S, Wehrens XH, Vest JA, et al. Beta-blockers restore calcium release channel function and improve cardiac muscle performance in human heart failure. Circulation 2003;107(19):2459–66.

70. Brixius K, Lu R, Boelck B, et al. Chronic treatment with carvedilol improves Ca(2+)-dependent ATP consumption in triton X-skinned fiber preparations

of human myocardium. J Pharmacol Exp Ther 2007;322(1):222–7.

71. Tamaki S, Sakata Y, Mano T, et al. Long-term beta-blocker therapy improves diastolic function even without the therapeutic effect on systolic function in patients with reduced ejection fraction. J Cardiol 2010;56(2):176–82.

72. Morita H, Suzuki G, Mishima T, et al. Effects of long-term monotherapy with metoprolol CR/XL on the progression of left ventricular dysfunction and remodeling in dogs with chronic heart failure. Cardiovasc Drugs Ther 2002;16(5):443–9.

73. Kobayashi M, Machida N, Mitsuishi M, et al. Beta-blocker improves survival, left ventricular function, and myocardial remodeling in hypertensive rats with diastolic heart failure. Am J Hypertens 2004; 17(12 Pt 1):1112–9.

74. Muller-Brunotte R, Kahan T, Lopez B, et al. Myocardial fibrosis and diastolic dysfunction in patients with hypertension: results from the Swedish Irbesartan Left Ventricular Hypertrophy Investigation versus Atenolol (SILVHIA). J Hypertens 2007; 25(9):1958–66.

75. The Beta-Blocker Heart Attack Trial. Beta-Blocker Heart Attack Study Group. JAMA 1981;246(18): 2073–4.

76. McMurray J, Kober L, Robertson M, et al. Antiarrhythmic effect of carvedilol after acute myocardial infarction: results of the Carvedilol Post-Infarct Survival Control in Left Ventricular Dysfunction (CAPRICORN) trial. J Am Coll Cardiol 2005;45(4): 525–30.

77. Lowes BD, Gilbert EM, Abraham WT, et al. Myocardial gene expression in dilated cardiomyopathy treated with beta-blocking agents. N Engl J Med 2002;346(18):1357–65.

78. Rathore SS, Curtis JP, Wang Y, et al. Association of serum digoxin concentration and outcomes in patients with heart failure. JAMA 2003;289(7):871–8.

79. Ribner HS, Plucinski DA, Hsieh AM, et al. Acute effects of digoxin on total systemic vascular resistance in congestive heart failure due to dilated cardiomyopathy: a hemodynamic-hormonal study. Am J Cardiol 1985;56(13):896–904.

80. Gheorghiade M. Digoxin therapy in chronic heart failure. Cardiovasc Drugs Ther 1997;11(Suppl 1): 279–83.

81. Gheorghiade M, Ferguson D. Digoxin. A neurohormonal modulator in heart failure? Circulation 1991; 84(5):2181–6.

82. Swedberg K, Bristow MR, Cohn JN, et al. Effects of sustained-release moxonidine, an imidazoline agonist, on plasma norepinephrine in patients with chronic heart failure. Circulation 2002;105(15):1797–803.

83. Cohn JN, Pfeffer MA, Rouleau J, et al. Adverse mortality effect of central sympathetic inhibition with sustained-release moxonidine in patients with heart failure (MOXCON). Eur J Heart Fail 2003; 5(5):659–67.

84. Skomedal T, Borthne K, Aass H, et al. Comparison between alpha-1 adrenoceptor-mediated and beta adrenoceptor-mediated inotropic components elicited by norepinephrine in failing human ventricular muscle. J Pharmacol Exp Ther 1997;280(2):721–9.

85. ALLHAT Officers and Coordinators for the ALLHAT Collaborative Research Group. The Antihypertensive and Lipid-Lowering Treatment to Prevent Heart Attack Trial. Major outcomes in high-risk hypertensive patients randomized to angiotensin-converting enzyme inhibitor or calcium channel blocker vs diuretic: The Antihypertensive and Lipid-Lowering Treatment to Prevent Heart Attack Trial (ALLHAT). JAMA 2002;288(23):2981–97.

86. Zhou J, Xu X, Liu JJ, et al. Angiotensin II receptors subtypes mediate diverse gene expression profile in adult hypertrophic cardiomyocytes. Clin Exp Pharmacol Physiol 2007;34(11):1191–8.

87. von Lueder TG, Sangaralingham SJ, Wang BH, et al. Renin-angiotensin blockade combined with natriuretic peptide system augmentation: novel therapeutic concepts to combat heart failure. Circ Heart Fail 2013;6(3):594–605.

88. Wehling M. Effects of aldosterone and mineralocorticoid receptor blockade on intracellular electrolytes. Heart Fail Rev 2005;10(1):39–46.

89. Sun Y. Myocardial repair/remodelling following infarction: roles of local factors. Cardiovasc Res 2009;81(3):482–90.

90. Lindpaintner K, Jin MW, Niedermaier N, et al. Cardiac angiotensinogen and its local activation in the isolated perfused beating heart. Circ Res 1990; 67(3):564–73.

91. Re R, Fallon JT, Dzau V, et al. Renin synthesis by canine aortic smooth muscle cells in culture. Life Sci 1982;30(1):99–106.

92. Serneri GG, Boddi M, Cecioni I, et al. Cardiac angiotensin II formation in the clinical course of heart failure and its relationship with left ventricular function. Circ Res 2001;88(9):961–8.

93. Dzau VJ. Implications of local angiotensin production in cardiovascular physiology and pharmacology. Am J Cardiol 1987;59(2):59A–65A.

94. Kato H, Suzuki H, Tajima S, et al. Angiotensin II stimulates collagen synthesis in cultured vascular smooth muscle cells. J Hypertens 1991;9(1):17–22.

95. Farquharson CA, Struthers AD. Aldosterone induces acute endothelial dysfunction in vivo in humans: evidence for an aldosterone-induced vasculopathy. Clin Sci 2002;103(4):425–31.

96. Kim S, Iwao H. Molecular and cellular mechanisms of angiotensin II-mediated cardiovascular and renal diseases. Pharmacol Rev 2000;52(1):11–34.

97. Sadoshima J, Izumo S. Molecular characterization of angiotensin II–induced hypertrophy of cardiac

myocytes and hyperplasia of cardiac fibroblasts. Critical role of the AT1 receptor subtype. Circ Res 1993;73(3):413–23.

98. Dostal DE, Baker KM. Angiotensin II stimulation of left ventricular hypertrophy in adult rat heart. Mediation by the AT1 receptor. Am J Hypertens 1992; 5(5 Pt 1):276–80.

99. Maruyama R, Hatta E, Yasuda K, et al. Angiotensin-converting enzyme-independent angiotensin formation in a human model of myocardial ischemia: modulation of norepinephrine release by angiotensin type 1 and angiotensin type 2 receptors. J Pharmacol Exp Ther 2000;294(1):248–54.

100. May CN, Yao ST, Booth LC, et al. Cardiac sympathoexcitation in heart failure. Auton Neurosci 2013;175(1–2):76–84.

101. Ramchandra R, Hood SG, Watson AM, et al. Central angiotensin type 1 receptor blockade decreases cardiac but not renal sympathetic nerve activity in heart failure. Hypertension 2012;59(3): 634–41.

102. McKinney CA, Fattah C, Loughrey CM, et al. Angiotensin-(1-7) and angiotensin-(1-9): function in cardiac and vascular remodelling. Clin Sci 2014; 126(12):815–27.

103. Regoli D, Plante GE, Gobeil F Jr. Impact of kinins in the treatment of cardiovascular diseases. Pharmacol Ther 2012;135(1):94–111.

104. Shearer F, Lang CC, Struthers AD. Renin-angiotensin-aldosterone system inhibitors in heart failure. Clin Pharmacol Ther 2013;94(4):459–67.

105. Packer M, Poole-Wilson PA, Armstrong PW, et al. Comparative effects of low and high doses of the angiotensin-converting enzyme inhibitor, lisinopril, on morbidity and mortality in chronic heart failure. ATLAS Study Group. Circulation 1999;100(23): 2312–8.

106. Konstam MA, Neaton JD, Dickstein K, et al. Effects of high-dose versus low-dose losartan on clinical outcomes in patients with heart failure (HEAAL study): a randomised, double-blind trial. Lancet 2009;374(9704):1840–8.

107. Pfeffer MA, Braunwald E, Moye LA, et al. Effect of captopril on mortality and morbidity in patients with left ventricular dysfunction after myocardial infarction. Results of the survival and ventricular enlargement trial. The SAVE Investigators. N Engl J Med 1992;327(10):669–77.

108. Naccarella F, Naccarelli GV, Maranga SS, et al. Do ACE inhibitors or angiotensin II antagonists reduce total mortality and arrhythmic mortality? A critical review of controlled clinical trials. Curr Opin Cardiol 2002;17(1):6–18.

109. Ruggenenti P, Perna A, Gherardi G, et al. Renoprotective properties of ACE-inhibition in non-diabetic nephropathies with non-nephrotic proteinuria. Lancet 1999;354(9176):359–64.

110. Roig E, Perez-Villa F, Morales M, et al. Clinical implications of increased plasma angiotensin II despite ACE inhibitor therapy in patients with congestive heart failure. Eur Heart J 2000;21(1):53–7.

111. Bomback AS, Klemmer PJ. The incidence and implications of aldosterone breakthrough. Nat Clin Pract Nephrol 2007;3(9):486–92.

112. Seva Pessoa B, van der Lubbe N, Verdonk K, et al. Key developments in renin-angiotensin-aldosterone system inhibition. Nat Rev Nephrol 2013;9(1):26–36.

113. Cohn JN, Tognoni G, Valsartan Heart Failure Trial Investigators. A randomized trial of the angiotensin-receptor blocker valsartan in chronic heart failure. N Engl J Med 2001;345(23):1667–75.

114. McMurray JJ, Ostergren J, Swedberg K, et al. Effects of candesartan in patients with chronic heart failure and reduced left-ventricular systolic function taking angiotensin-converting-enzyme inhibitors: the CHARM-Added trial. Lancet 2003; 362(9386):767–71.

115. Phillips CO, Kashani A, Ko DK, et al. Adverse effects of combination angiotensin II receptor blockers plus angiotensin-converting enzyme inhibitors for left ventricular dysfunction: a quantitative review of data from randomized clinical trials. Arch Intern Med 2007;167(18):1930–6.

116. Gheorghiade M, Bohm M, Greene SJ, et al. Effect of aliskiren on postdischarge mortality and heart failure readmissions among patients hospitalized for heart failure: the ASTRONAUT randomized trial. JAMA 2013;309(11):1125–35.

117. Krum H, Massie B, Abraham WT, et al. Direct renin inhibition in addition to or as an alternative to angiotensin converting enzyme inhibition in patients with chronic systolic heart failure: rationale and design of the Aliskiren Trial to Minimize OutcomeS in Patients with HEart failuRE (ATMOSPHERE) study. Eur J Heart Fail 2011;13(1):107–14.

118. Potter LR, Abbey-Hosch S, Dickey DM. Natriuretic peptides, their receptors, and cyclic guanosine monophosphate-dependent signaling functions. Endocr Rev 2006;27(1):47–72.

119. Richards AM, Lainchbury JG, Troughton RW, et al. Clinical applications of B-type natriuretic peptides. Trends Endocrinol Metab 2004;15(4):170–4.

120. Del Ry S. C-type natriuretic peptide: a new cardiac mediator. Peptides 2013;40:93–8.

121. Wada A, Tsutamoto T, Matsuda Y, et al. Cardiorenal and neurohumoral effects of endogenous atrial natriuretic peptide in dogs with severe congestive heart failure using a specific antagonist for guanylate cyclase-coupled receptors. Circulation 1994; 89(5):2232–40.

122. Kuhn M. Structure, regulation, and function of mammalian membrane guanylyl cyclase receptors, with a focus on guanylyl cyclase-A. Circ Res 2003; 93(8):700–9.

123. Tamura N, Ogawa Y, Chusho H, et al. Cardiac fibrosis in mice lacking brain natriuretic peptide. Proc Natl Acad Sci U S A 2000;97(8):4239–44.

124. Kishimoto I, Rossi K, Garbers DL. A genetic model provides evidence that the receptor for atrial natriuretic peptide (guanylyl cyclase-A) inhibits cardiac ventricular myocyte hypertrophy. Proc Natl Acad Sci U S A 2001;98(5):2703–6.

125. Soeki T, Kishimoto I, Okumura H, et al. C-type natriuretic peptide, a novel antifibrotic and antihypertrophic agent, prevents cardiac remodeling after myocardial infarction. J Am Coll Cardiol 2005;45(4):608–16.

126. O'Connor CM, Starling RC, Hernandez AF, et al. Effect of nesiritide in patients with acute decompensated heart failure. N Engl J Med 2011;365(1):32–43.

127. Mangiafico S, Costello-Boerrigter LC, Andersen IA, et al. Neutral endopeptidase inhibition and the natriuretic peptide system: an evolving strategy in cardiovascular therapeutics. Eur Heart J 2013;34(12):886–893c.

128. Kostis JB, Packer M, Black HR, et al. Omapatrilat and enalapril in patients with hypertension: the Omapatrilat Cardiovascular Treatment vs. Enalapril (OCTAVE) trial. Am J Hypertens 2004;17(2):103–11.

129. McMurray JJ, Packer M, Desai AS, et al. Dual angiotensin receptor and neprilysin inhibition as an alternative to angiotensin-converting enzyme inhibition in patients with chronic systolic heart failure: rationale for and design of the Prospective comparison of ARNI with ACEI to Determine Impact on Global Mortality and morbidity in Heart Failure trial (PARADIGM-HF). Eur J Heart Fail 2013;15(9):1062–73.

130. Goldsmith SR, Francis GS, Cowley AW Jr, et al. Increased plasma arginine vasopressin levels in patients with congestive heart failure. J Am Coll Cardiol 1983;1(6):1385–90.

131. Hupf H, Grimm D, Riegger GA, et al. Evidence for a vasopressin system in the rat heart. Circ Res 1999; 84(3):365–70.

132. Li X, Chan TO, Myers V, et al. Controlled and cardiac-restricted overexpression of the arginine vasopressin V1A receptor causes reversible left ventricular dysfunction through Galphaq-mediated cell signaling. Circulation 2011;124(5): 572–81.

133. Gheorghiade M, Konstam MA, Burnett JC Jr, et al. Short-term clinical effects of tolvaptan, an oral vasopressin antagonist, in patients hospitalized for heart failure: the EVEREST Clinical Status Trials. JAMA 2007;297(12):1332–43.

134. Schrier RW, Gross P, Gheorghiade M, et al. Tolvaptan, a selective oral vasopressin V2-receptor antagonist, for hyponatremia. N Engl J Med 2006;355(20): 2099–112.

135. Movassagh M, Choy MK, Knowles DA, et al. Distinct epigenomic features in end-stage failing human hearts. Circulation 2011;124(22):2411–22.

136. Papait R, Greco C, Kunderfranco P, et al. Epigenetics: a new mechanism of regulation of heart failure? Basic Res Cardiol 2013;108(4):361.

137. Anand P, Brown JD, Lin CY, et al. BET bromodomains mediate transcriptional pause release in heart failure. Cell 2013;154(3):569–82.

138. Kumarswamy R, Thum T. Non-coding RNAs in cardiac remodeling and heart failure. Circ Res 2013; 113(6):676–89.

Mineralcorticoid Antagonists in Heart Failure

Emilia D'Elia, MD[a,b], Henry Krum, MBBS, PhD, FRACP, FCSANZ, FESC[c],*

KEYWORDS

- Mineralcorticoid receptor agonists - Heart failure - Aldosterone

KEY POINTS

- Aldosterone is the most important corticosteroid hormone in the human body responsible for several critical pathophysiological contributions to the heart failure (HF) syndrome.
- Mineralcorticoid receptor agonists (MRAs) have been documented to be effective in opposing these adverse effects of aldosterone in HF, favoring reduction of congestion, hemodynamic improvement, decrease in vasoconstriction, and abrogation of pathologic cardiac fibrosis.
- With their antiremodeling effects, these drugs seems to be powerful in HF both early after myocardial infarction and in established disease.
- MRAs are recommended for all HF patients with persisting symptoms (New York Heart Association class II-IV) and a left ventricular ejection fraction no more than 35% despite treatment with an angiotensin-converting enzyme inhibitor and a beta-blocker, to reduce the risk of re-hospitalization and the risk of premature death (I-A recommendation).
- Further areas currently being explored for MRAs include their use in patients with heart failure with preserved ejection fraction (HFPEF) and early after MI.
- Renal function and serum potassium should be carefully monitored, particularly with the introduction of MRA.

INTRODUCTION

Heart failure (HF) is a syndrome characterized by the activation of several neurohormonal mechanisms initially focused on maintaining an adequate peripheral perfusion, but potentially causing counterproductive physiopatological alterations such as hydrosaline retention, peripheral vasoconstriction, and myocyte degeneration/hypertrophy.[1,2] The renin angiotensin aldosterone system (RAAS) and autonomic nervous system are important and interdependent mechanisms contributing to these pathophysiological responses. Both tissue and peripheral RAAS activation induce production of

angiotensin II, which is one of the more powerful vasoconstrictive peptide hormones in the body.[3] RAAS activation takes place in vascular, renal, and cardiac structures, favoring the phenomenon of left ventricular remodeling: angiotensin II facilitates myocyte growth and represents a stimulus for norepinephrine release. The SOLVD (Studies of Left Ventricular Dysfunction) study demonstrated a significant reduction in left ventricular dimensions in HF patients treated with an angiotensin-converting enzyme (ACE) inhibitor (enalapril), likely due not only to a decrease in afterload, but also to blockade of local activation of myocardial RAAS.[4] Many other clinical trials[5–7] support the relevance

a Cardiovascular Department, Papa Giovanni XXIII Hospital, Piazza OMS 1, Bergamo 24127, Italy; b University of Pavia, Piazzale Golgi 1, Pavia 27100, Italy; c Department of Epidemiology & Preventive Medicine, Centre of Cardiovascular Research & Education (CCRE) in Therapeutics, Alfred Hospital, Monash University, Commercial Road, Melbourne, Victoria 3004, Australia
* Corresponding author.
E-mail address: henry.krum@monash.edu

Heart Failure Clin 10 (2014) 559–564
http://dx.doi.org/10.1016/j.hfc.2014.07.003
1551-7136/14/$ – see front matter © 2014 Elsevier Inc. All rights reserved.

of these system interactions in HF patients, focusing on the role of ACE inhibitors in improving symptoms and reducing mortality.

ROLE OF ALDOSTERONE IN HF

ACE inhibitors can cause an initial reduction of plasma angiotensin II and aldosterone levels, although over the long term, their efficacy is lowered, probably because of aldosterone escape, a phenomenon first observed in hypertensive patients when high-dose ACE inhibitors (captopril) were associated with an increase rather than decrease in aldosterone levels.[8,9] With prolonged blockade of the ACE enzyme, it is reasonable to assume that other mechanisms (ie, increases in adrenocorticotrophin [ACTH], endothelin, or intracellular electrolytes) become more critical for aldosterone release. In the HF syndrome, plasma aldosterone levels are correlated with worsening

of HF and increased mortality, as has been demonstrated in the CONSENSUS (Cooperative North Scandinavian Enalapril Survival Study) trial.[10]

Aldosterone is the most powerful corticosteroid hormone in the human body. It is responsible for salt and water balance, and its augmented production confers a critical negative role in the HF setting, where mineralcorticoid receptors (MR) are overexpressed.[11]

Aldosterone activation confers negative effects at several different levels (**Figs. 1** and **2**)[12]:

- At the renal distal tubule, it causes sodium retention and loss of potassium and magnesium. The consequent extravascular volume expansion determines volume overload and venous pressure increase, worsening edema and congestion, with further RAAS activation.
- At the myocardial level, it favors myocyte fibrosis, increased oxygen demand, and

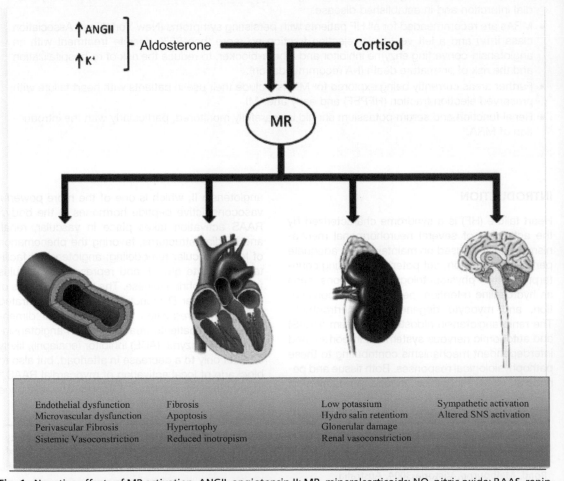

Endothelial dysfunction	Fibrosis	Low potassium	Sympathetic activation
Microvascular dysfunction	Apoptosis	Hydro salin retentiom	Altered SNS activation
Perivascular Fibrosis	Hyperrtophy	Glonerular damage	
Sistemic Vasoconstriction	Reduced inotropism	Renal vasoconstriction	

Fig. 1. Negative effects of MR activation. ANGII, angiotensin II; MR, mineralcorticoids; NO, nitric oxide; RAAS, renin-angiotensin-aldosterone system; SNS, sympathetic nervous system. (*Adapted from* Albaghdadi M, Gheorghiade M, Pitt B. Mineralocorticoid receptor antagonism: therapeutic potential in acute heart failure syndromes. Eur Heart J 2011;32:2627; with permission.)

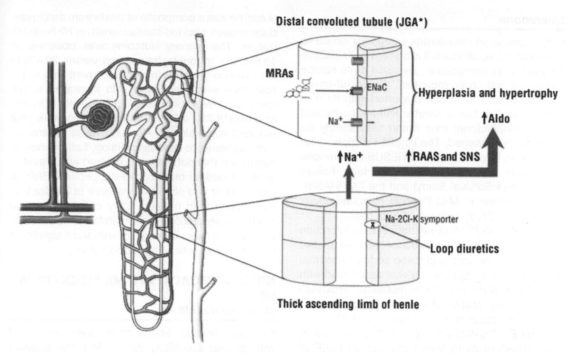

Fig. 2. Resistance to diuretics and antialdosterone effects of MRAs. Sodium increase causes hyperplasia and hypertrophy at distal tubule level with activation of RAAS and SNS and consequently increase of aldosterone plasma levels. In HF patients, MRA favor natriuresis. * JGA, juxtaglomerular apparatus. (*Adapted from* Albaghdadi M, Gheorghiade M, Pitt B. Mineralocorticoid receptor antagonism: therapeutic potential in acute heart failure syndromes. Eur Heart J 2011;32:2632; with permission.)

pathologic myocardial collagen production; all of these effects contribute to ventricular stiffness and diastolic dysfunction.

- At the vascular level, it causes vasoconstriction, afterload increase, and endothelial dysfunction; spironolactone, an MR antagonist (MRA), improves endothelial function in HF patients already treated with ACE inhibitors.[13]
- At the hemocoagulative level, it favors fibrinolysis, causing an increase in endothelial plasminogen activator inhibitor.
- At the neurohormonal level, it has an indirect sympathomimetic action, enhancing catecholamine effect and inhibiting norephinephrine reuptake.

MRAS IN HF CLINICAL TRIALS
Spironolactone

In the Randomized Aldactone Evaluation Study (RALES), a population of 1663 systolic HF patients with New York Heart Association (NHYA) class III to IV symptoms receiving standard medical therapy was randomized to receive spironolactone (25 mg daily) or placebo. Spironolactone was associated with a significant mortality (-30%, P<.001) and rehospitalization reduction.[14]

Because of the adverse effects of the drug (gynecomastia, lightheadedness, high serum potassium levels), new clinical trials have been performed to assess the efficacy of MRAs with fewer off-target effects.

Canrenone

Canrenone is the principal active metabolite of spironolactone and a competitive inhibitor of the MR. In the AREA IN-CHF 21 (Antiremodeling Effect of Aldosterone Receptors Blockade with Canrenone in Mild Heart Failure) trial, canrenone versus placebo was tested in patients with mild HF (NHYA class II symptoms, left ventricular ejection fraction [LVEF] <45%) already on ACE inhibitors, beta-blockers, and digitalis.[15] The primary endpoint of diastolic ventricular diameter reduction was not achieved, but at 9 months follow-up canrenone was associated with an improvement in LVEF, a reduction in rehospitalization for HF, and a reduction of the combined endpoint of mortality and rehospitalization. Gynecomastia and higher potassium levels were not significantly increased as adverse effects, but renal function worsened with canrenone versus placebo (creatinine >2.5 mg/dL 2.2% vs 0.4% respectively, $P = .01$).

Eplerenone

Eplerenone is an aldosterone antagonist similar to spironolactone, although it is much more selective for the MR in comparison. Because of its scarce affinity to estrogen receptors, fewer off-target adverse effects have been reported with its use. Furthermore, it has a shorter half-life compared with spironolactone; thus it can theoretically be more easily managed. The largest HF trials using eplerenone have been the EPHESUS (Eplerenone Post-Acute Myocardial Infarction Heart Failure Efficacy and Survival Study) and the EMPHASIS-HF (Eplerenone in Mild Patients Hospitalizations and Survival Study in Heart Failure) trials.[16,17]

In EPHESUS,[16] 6632 postmyocardial infarction (MI) patients with LVEF less than 40% were treated with eplerenone versus placebo added to optimal medical therapy. Eplerenone was associated with a significant reduction in total mortality, cardiovascular mortality, and sudden cardiac death (respectively, a reduction of 15%, 17%, and 21%).

In the EMPHASIS-HF trial,[17] 2737 patients with mild (NYHA class II) symptoms and an LVEF of no more than 35% were randomized to receive eplerenone (up to 50 mg daily) or placebo, in addition to recommended therapy. The primary outcome was a composite of death from cardiovascular causes or hospitalization for heart failure. The trial was stopped prematurely after a median follow-up period of 21 months. The primary outcome occurred in 18.3% of patients in the eplerenone group as compared with 25.9% in the placebo group ($P<.001$). Other interesting subanalyses of the EMPHASIS-HF trials documented the efficacy of eplerenone in high-risk patients, such as in the elderly, diabetics, patients with renal insufficiency and low blood pressure.[18,19]

MRAS IN HF WITH PRESERVED EJECTION FRACTION (HFPEF)

As alluded to previously, activation of aldosterone appears to make an important contribution to the progression of diastolic dysfunction via systemic hypertension, myocyte hypertrophy, and especially pathologic deposition of extracellular matrix material within the myocardium. Several small studies of MRAs have suggested beneficial effects of MRAs on these processes in patients with HFPEF. The recently published TOPCAT (Treatment of Preserved Cardiac Function Heart Failure with an Aldosterone Antagonist) study[20] was a randomized, double-blind trial of 3445 patients with symptomatic heart failure and an LVEF of greater than 45%. Patients were randomized to receive either spironolactone (15–45 mg daily) or placebo. The primary

outcome was a composite of death from cardiovascular causes, aborted cardiac arrest, or HF hospitalization. The primary outcome was observed in 18.6% the spironolactone group versus 20.4% in the placebo group, $P = .14$. Treatment with spironolactone was associated with increased serum creatinine levels and a doubling of the rate of hyperkalemia (18.7%, vs 9.1% in the placebo group) but reduced hypokalemia. Although these topline results appeared to be disappointing, further analysis suggested that patients who entered with elevated levels of plasma brain natriuretic peptide (BNP) (a more robust and objective measure of LV diastolic dysfunction than meeting entry criteria based on an HF hospitalization), demonstrated a much higher incidence of major outcome events and a significant reduction in events with spironolactone.

NOVEL APPROACHES TO MR BLOCKADE IN HF
Nonsteroidal MRAs

New nonsteroidal MRAs have been developed with greater specificity for the MR and putative greater affinity for cardiac versus renal MR. In theory, this should lead to fewer off-target effects and less hyperkalemia than conventional MRAs. BAY 94–8862 is the most advanced nonsteroidal MRA in clinical development. It has been studied in patients with low EF HF and mild-to-moderate chronic kidney disease (CKD).[21] The agent was associated with smaller increases in serum potassium levels versus spironolactone, with less renal impairment despite similar decreases in plasma BNP. A large phase 2B minerAlocorticoid Receptor Antagonist Tolerability Study-Heart Failure (ARTS-HF) is currently ongoing with BAY 94–8862 in low LVEF HF patients with mild renal impairment and diabetes or moderate renal impairment.

Aldosterone Synthase Inhibitors

Aldosterone synthase is the final enzyme involved in the pathway of endogenous aldosterone production. Thus, aldosterone synthase inhibition (ASI) should directly reduce circulating aldosterone levels (rather than increase, as observed with MRAs). LCI699 is an ASI recently studied in patients with systemic hypertension. Reductions in blood pressure (BP) were similar to those observed with eplerenone at approved BP-lowering doses.[22] However, ASI may also result in inhibition of cortisol release. Adrenocorticotropic hormone stimulation testing suggested suppression of cortisol in patients receiving LCI699 at BP-lowering doses. In HF, a disorder associated with enhanced catabolism, a modest degree of cortisol inhibition may be advantageous rather than deleterious.

However, it is uncertain whether further development of this agent or other ASIs will be continued.

SUMMARY

Aldosterone is the most important corticosteroid hormone in the human body, responsible for several critical pathophysiological contributions to the HF syndrome. MRAs have been documented to be effective in opposing these adverse effects of aldosterone in HF, favoring reduction of congestion, hemodynamic improvement, decreased in vasoconstriction, and abrogation of pathologic cardiac fibrosis. With their antiremodeling effects, these drugs seem to be powerful in HF both early after MI and in established disease. According to the most recent European Society of Cardiology (ESC) guidelines for the diagnosis and treatment of HF,[23] MRAs are recommended for all HF patients with persisting symptoms (NYHA class II-IV) and an LVEF of no more than 35% despite treatment with an ACE inhibitor and a beta-blocker, to reduce the risk of re-hospitalization and the risk of premature death (I-A recommendation). Further areas currently being explored for MRAs include in patients with HFPEF and very early after MI.

REFERENCES

1. Francis GS, Goldsmith SR, Levine BT, et al. The neurohumoral axis in congestive heart failure. Ann Intern Med 1984;101:370–7.
2. Gavazzi A. Fisiopatologia. In: Gavazzi A, editor. Lo scompenso cardiaco. Milano (Italy): Scripta Manent snc Ed; 2002. p. 25–50.
3. Dzau VJ, Gibbson GH. Autocrine–paracrine mechanisms of vascular myocytes in hypertension. Am J Cardiol 1987;60:991.
4. Konstam MA, Rousseau MF, Kronenberg MW, et al. Effects of angiotensin converting enzyme inhibitor, enalapril, on long-term progression of left ventricular dysfunction in patients with heart failure. Circulation 1992;86:431–8.
5. Swedberg K, Eneroth P, Krjekshus J, et al. Hormones regulating cardiovascular function in patients with severe congestive heart failure and their relation to mortality. Circulation 1990;82:1730–6.
6. Francis GS, Cohn JN, Johnson G, et al. Plasma norepinephrine, plasma renin activity, and congestive heart failure. Relations to survival and the effects of therapy in V-HeFT II. The V-HeFT VA Cooperative Studies Group. Circulation 1993;87(Suppl VI): VI-40–8.
7. Benedict CR, Weiner DH, Johnstone DE, et al. Comparative neurohormonal responses in patients with preserved and impaired left ventricular ejection fraction: results of the studies of left ventricular dysfunction (SOLVD) registry. J Am Coll Cardiol 1993;22(Suppl A):146A–53A.
8. Staessen J, Lijnen P, Fagard R, et al. Rise in plasma concentration of aldosterone during long-term angiotensin II suppression. J Endocrinol 1981;91:457–65.
9. Borghi C, Boschi S, Ambrosioni E, et al. Evidence of a partial escape of renin-angiotensin-aldosterone blockade in patients with acute myocardial infarction treated with ACE-inhibitors. J Clin Pharmacol 1993; 33:40–5.
10. Effects of enalapril on mortality in severe congestive heart failure: results of the Cooperative North Scandinavian Enalapril Survival Study (CONSENSUS). The CONSENSUS Trial Study Group. N Engl J Med 1987;316:1429–35.
11. Greco C, Castelli G, Crea F, et al. Nuove evidenze sull'impiego degli antialdosteronici nella disfunzione ventricolare sinistra: spironolattone ed eplerenone. Dal postinfarto allo scompenso cardiaco. G Ital Cardiol 2012;13:809–16.
12. Albaghdadi M, Gheorghiade M, Pitt B. Mineralocorticoid receptor antagonism: therapeutic potential in acute heart failure syndromes. Eur Heart J 2011; 32:2626–33.
13. Macdonald JE, Kennedy N, Struthers AD. Effects of spironolactone on endothelial function, vascular angiotensin converting enzyme activity, and other prognostic markers in patients with mild heart failure already taking optimal treatment. Heart 2004;90: 765–70.
14. Pitt B, Zannad F, Remme W, et al. The effect of spironolactone on morbidity and mortality in patients with severe heart failure. N Engl J Med 1999;341: 709–17.
15. Boccanelli A, Mureddu GF, Cacciatore G, et al. on behalf of AREA IN-CHF Investigators. Antiremodeling effect of canrenone in patients with mild chronic heart failure (AREA IN-CHF study): final results. Eur J Heart Fail 2009;11:68–76.
16. Pitt B, Remme W, Zannad F, et al, for the Eplerenone Post-acute Myocardial Infarction Efficacy and survival Study Investigators. Eplerenone, a selective aldosterone blocker, in patients with left ventricular dysfunction after myocardial infarction. N Engl J Med 2003;348:1309–21.
17. Zannad F, McMurray JJ, Krum H, et al. Eplerenone in patients with systolic heart failure and mild symptoms. N Engl J Med 2011;364:11–21.
18. Krum H, Shi H, Pitt B, et al. Clinical benefit of eplerenone in patients with mild symptoms of systolic heart failure already receiving optimal best practice background drug therapy: analysis of the EMPHASIS-HF study. Circ Heart Fail 2013;6(4):711–8.
19. Rogers JK, McMurray JJ, Pocock SJ, et al. Eplerenone in patients with systolic heart failure and mild symptoms: analysis of repeat hospitalizations. Circulation 2012;126:2317–23.

20. Pitt B, Pfeffer MA, Assmann SF, et al. TOPCAT investigators. Spironolactone for heart failure with preserved ejection fraction. N Engl J Med 2014;370:1383–92.

21. Pitt B, Kober L, Ponikowski P, et al. Safety and tolerability of the novel non-steroidal mineralocorticoid receptor antagonist BAY 94-8862 in patients with chronic heart failure and mild or moderate chronic kidney disease: a randomized, double-blind trial. Eur Heart J 2013;34:2453–63.

22. Calhoun DA, White WB, Krum H, et al. Effects of a novel aldosterone synthase inhibitor for treatment of primary hypertension: results of a randomized, double-blind, placebo- and active-controlled phase 2 trial. Circulation 2011;124:1945–55.

23. McMurray JJ, Adamopoulos S, Anker SD, et al. ESC Guidelines for the diagnosis and treatment of acute and chronic heart failure 2012. Eur Heart J 2012;33: 1787–847.

Current Perspectives on Hydralazine and Nitrate Therapies in Heart Failure

Robert T. Cole, MD*, Divya Gupta, MD,
Javed Butler, MD, MPH

KEYWORDS

• Hydralazine • Nitrates • Congestive heart failure • Vasodilators

KEY POINTS

- Hydralazine/nitrate combination therapy has been proved effective in black heart failure (HF) patients, yet these drugs are markedly underused in this population.
- The true benefit of hydralazine/nitrate combination therapy may result from the drugs' effects on the nitroso-redox balance as opposed to their individual hemodynamics effects.
- Retrospective studies suggest the benefit of hydralazine and nitrate combination therapy may be greater in certain subpopulations of HF, including women and the elderly.
- Other HF therapies (eg, angiotensin-converting enzyme inhibitors [ACEIs]) have antioxidant effects similar to hydralazine; these alternative antioxidant agents might be substituted for hydralazine, obviating a thrice-a-day drug with many adverse side effects.

INTRODUCTION

For many decades, the treatment of HF centered around the use of digitalis, diuretics, and archaic rituals, such as rotating tourniquets.[1,2] Although these interventions improved symptoms, there was no conclusive evidence that any of them had a significant effect on patient survival. In the 1970s, however, a new concept emerged: that pharmacologic reduction in systemic vascular resistance may improve cardiac performance and potentially improve outcomes for patients with HF.[3] This led to many physiologic and clinical studies of vasodilators in HF.[4] Early successes with intravenous vasodilators like sodium nitroprusside[5,6] gave way to clinical trials with various oral agents, including the combination of hydralazine and isosorbide dinitrate (H+ISDN). This combination mimics the effects of sodium nitroprusside (ie, balanced arterial and venous dilatation), leading to reductions in afterload and preload, respectively.[7,8] Initial success in smaller trials led to several randomized controlled clinical trials (**Table 1**) that ultimately established H+ISDN as a mainstay of therapy for many patients with HF. Yet despite the benefits of H+ISDN shown in clinical trials, there remains ongoing discussion on several pertinent issues, including (1) Is the benefit of H+ISDN rooted in pure hemodynamic effects versus its role in maintaining the nitroso-redox balance? (2) Which populations of HF patients should receive H+ISDN? (ie, Is the benefit limited to specific HF patients only?) (3) Are alternative agents as effective as hydralazine when combined with ISDN? and (4) Why do so few eligible patients receive this therapy? This article discusses what is currently known about H+ISDN and reviews these ongoing topics of debate.

Conflict of Interest: None.
Division of Cardiology, Emory University, 1365 Clifton Road Northeast, Atlanta, GA 30322, USA
* Corresponding author. Center for Heart Failure Therapy, Emory University Hospital, 1365 Clifton Road Northeast, Suite A1214, Atlanta, GA 30322.
E-mail address: rtcole@emory.edu

Heart Failure Clin 10 (2014) 565–576
http://dx.doi.org/10.1016/j.hfc.2014.07.001
1551-7136/14/$ – see front matter © 2014 Elsevier Inc. All rights reserved.

Table 1
Randomized controlled trials of hydralazine + isosorbide dinitrate in heart failure

Study	Target Dose of H + ISDN	Comparator	N	Patients	Major Endpoints	Results	Notable
V-HeFT I	300 mg Hydral 160 mg ISDN	• Prazosin 20 mg • Placebo	642	• All male symptomatic CHF • EF <45% or dilated • Background digoxin and diuretics	• Mortality • Change in EF	• H+ISDN reduced mortality (RRR) by 34% at 2 y (P<.028) compared with placebo • Overall mortality reduction of marginal significance • H+ISDN improved EF compared with placebo	Only 55% of patients target dose at 6 mo
V-HeFT II	300 mg Hydral 160 mg ISDN	Enalapril 20 mg	804	• All male • Symptomatic CHF • EF <45% or dilated • Background digoxin and diuretics	• Mortality • Exercise tolerance • Change in EF • Hospitalization	• No significant difference in overall mortality • Enalapril superior for mortality at 2 y (18% vs 25%, P = .018) • H+ISDN superior for EF at 13 wk, but no difference overall (both improved EF) • H+ISDN superior for exercise capacity improvement • No difference in hospitalization rates	Approximately 30% discontinued H+ISDN
A-HeFT	225 mg Hydral 120 mg ISDN	Placebo	1050	• All African American • NYHA III/IV • EF <35% or <45% + dilated • Background ACEI, BB, aldosterone antagonists	• Composite score of morality + CHF hospitalization + QOL • Individual components of composite (secondary endpoints)	• H+ISDN reduced mortality (RRR) by 43% compared with placebo • Composite score significantly better in H+ISDN • Fewer CHF hospitalizations in H+ISDN	47% of H+ISDN had headaches and 29% reported dizziness 68% of patients achieved target dose of H+ISDN

Abbreviations: BB, β-blockers; CHF, congestive HF; Hydral, hydralazine; QOL, quality of life; RRR, relative risk reduction.

HISTORICAL PERSPECTIVES: THE RANDOMIZED CONTROLLED CLINICAL TRIALS OF H+ISDN

Since the early hemodynamic studies by Massie and colleagues and Pierpont and colleagues,[7,8] there have been 3 large-scale, randomized clinical trials of H+ISDN in HF, spanning 3 decades. Knowledge of these trials is critical to understanding the role of H+ISDN in practice today.

Vasodilators-Heart Failure Trial I—1986

The evolution of H+ISDN finds its roots in the first major randomized placebo-controlled clinical trial in HF: the Vasodilator-Heart Failure Trial (V-HeFT I), published approximately 30 years ago.[9] This study randomized 642 men with systolic dysfunction in the Veterans Affairs (VA) hospital system to 1 of 3 treatments: H+ISDN (target total daily dose of 300 mg hydralazine and 160 mg ISDN), prazosin, or placebo. At enrollment patients were on background therapy with digoxin and diuretics, the only available therapies for HF at the time. The use of H+ISDN compared with placebo was associated with a relative reduction in the risk of death by 34% at a prespecified 2-year time-point (P<.028). The relative mortality reduction of 12% throughout the overall study period was of marginal statistical significance. H+ISDN was also associated with improvements in ejection fraction (EF) compared with placebo.[9] Side effects were significant likely as a result of the high target doses of these agents, and only 55% of patients were taking the target doses 6 months into enrollment. Nonetheless, for the first time in the modern era, there was hope that this new combination could have an impact on the growing population of dying HF patients.

Vasodilator-Heart Failure II—1991

With the success exhibited in V-HeFT I, investigators decided to compare H+ISDN to the "new kids on the block," the ACEI in V-HeFT II.[10] This trial randomized 804 male patients in the VA health system with systolic dysfunction to either H+ISDN (target dose 300 mg hydralazine/160 mg ISDN total daily) or enalapril (20 mg daily). Similar to V-HeFT I, patients were on background therapy with digoxin and diuretics at enrollment. Mortality in the enalapril arm was statistically better compared with H+ISDN at the prespecified 2-year endpoint (18% vs 25%, P = .018); however, this was no longer significant when assessed in the overall study period (P = .08). Worth noting is that, despite the suggestion of greater mortality benefit with ACEI therapy, the use of H+ISDN was associated with greater improvements in exercise tolerance (peak oxygen consumption) and EF compared with enalapril.[10] Also, in contrast to other ACEI studies, the major mortality benefit of enalapril was a reduction in sudden death (prior studies showed primarily reduction in pump failure[11]). This was the first sign that ACEIs could have alternative mechanisms of action beyond pure vasodilation, and the investigators hypothesize there may be a potential role for combined therapy with both ACEIs and H+ISDN.

African-American Heart Failure Trial—2004

Retrospective analysis of the V-HeFT I and II studies suggested there might be a race-dependent response to H+ISDN therapy (**Fig. 1**).[12] Black patients seemed to derive substantial benefit, whereas white patients did not. The African-American Heart Failure Trial (A-HeFT) sought to further assess whether black patients with systolic HF truly derive such a considerable mortality

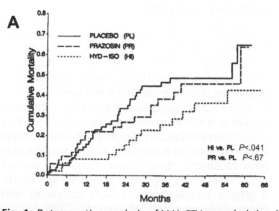

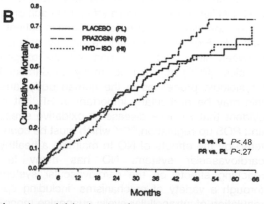

Fig. 1. Retrospective analysis of V-HeFT I revealed that black patients (*A*) had a significant improvement in mortality with H+ISDN compared with placebo, whereas white patients (*B*) did not. (*From* Carson P, Ziesche S, Johnson G, et al. Racial differences in response to therapy for heart failure: analysis of the vasodilator-heart failure trials. Vasodilator-Heart Failure Trial Study Group. J Card Fail 1999;5(3):178–87; with permission.)

benefit on top of standard medical therapy in the modern era (β-blockers, ACEIs, aldosterone blockers, and so forth).[13] The trial enrolled 1050 black patients with reduced EF and New York Heart Association (NYHA) III or IV symptoms despite optimal medical therapy. Patients were randomized to H+ISDN (target total daily doses of hydralazine 225 mg/isosorbide dinitrate [ISDN] 120 mg) or placebo, and the primary outcome was a weighted composite score of death, HF hospitalization, and change in quality of life. The trial was terminated early due to a clear, significant mortality benefit in the treatment arm compared with placebo (relative risk reduction of 43%, absolute reduction 4%; $P = .01$). In addition, there was significant improvement in each of the components of the composite score.[13] In light of these results, the Food and Drug Administration (FDA) later approved BiDil (a single pill formulation of H+ISDN) specifically for treatment of HF in African Americans. This marked the first time the FDA had ever approved a drug for one specific race.

THE H+ISDN BENEFIT: HEMODYNAMIC EFFECTS OR FUNDAMENTAL PATHOPHYSIOLOGY?

Although the combination of H+ISDN was initially used for the beneficial hemodynamic effects of the individual drugs, there is ongoing speculation that the improvement in outcomes with H+ISDN may be unrelated to their effects on hemodynamics. Critics of the hemodynamic theory argue that there have been countless other vasodilator drugs that improve hemodynamics in HF,[14–17] but they do not favorably affect outcomes in a fashion similar to H+ISDN.[18] In addition, the effects on preload/afterload with H+ISDN are not expected to preferentially benefit one race over the other.

The emerging theory on the true benefit of H+ISDN lies in the favorable effects of each drug on the so-called nitroso-redox balance in patients with HF (**Fig. 2**). Maintaining a healthy balance between nitric oxide (NO) and reactive oxygen species (ROS) is vital to many fundamental physiologic processes in the human body, and this may be particularly important in HF.[19] It is evident that HF is a disease of oxidative stress and ROS up-regulation,[20–22] which must be countered by the effects of NO to maintain a healthy cardiovascular system. NO has many far-reaching effects on the cardiovascular system through a variety of mechanisms, including up-regulation of intracellular cyclic guanosine monophosphate (cGMP) via guanylyl cyclase activation, S-nitrosylation of effector proteins leading to downstream activation of the myocyte ryanodine

receptor, and the formation of peroxynitrite, a toxic free radical with numerous deleterious effects, to name a few.[19,23–29] These fundamental pathophysiologic effects lead to a variety of downstream benefits, including enhanced endothelial function, improved cardiac contractility, and inhibition of adverse cardiac remodeling.[23,25,26,30–33]

The union of hydralazine with ISDN is a particularly fortuitous one, because in addition to their balanced vasodilatory effects, both drugs seem to have favorable effects on the nitroso-redox balance. Although ISDN is an NO donor and serves to augment NO availability, hydralazine has been shown to have antioxidant properties as a potent free radical scavenger.[34–37] The addition of hydralazine to organic nitrates has been shown historically to reduce the development of nitrate tolerance through the inhibition of ROS production[37,38] and, more recently, to restore impaired excitation-contraction coupling associated with nitroso-redox imbalance.[39] In light of these findings, it is reasonable to speculate that the benefits of H+ISDN may be related to maintenance of the nitroso-redox balance (and therefore inhibition of nitrate tolerance) instead of pure hemodynamic effects. This could also explain the preferential benefit seen in African American patients compared with whites, because black patients have been shown to have much greater impairment in NO-mediated processes.[4] This concept has not been fully validated and remains speculative at this time. The H+ISDN combination has never been compared directly to the individual components alone in the clinical trial setting nor has the combination of ISDN with alternative antioxidant agents been assessed for efficacy in HF.

WHO SHOULD TAKE HYDRALAZINE? DOES RACE MATTER? DOES GENDER MATTER? DOES AGE MATTER?
Race and H+ISDN

The beneficial effects of H+ISDN in African Americans with systolic HF has been clearly established in a large-scale clinical trial, A-HeFT, as discussed previously. Although retrospective analyses of the V-HeFT I/II trials suggested there was no mortality benefit to H+ISDN in nonblack patients,[12] this has never been validated in a large-scale clinical trial in the modern era of β-blockers, ACEIs, and aldosterone blockade. Nonetheless, there are several hypotheses as to why black patients might derive a greater benefit from H+ISDN compared with comparable nonblack HF patients. Chief among these is that black patients repeatedly have been shown to have significant impairments in several NO-mediated mechanisms. For example, in a

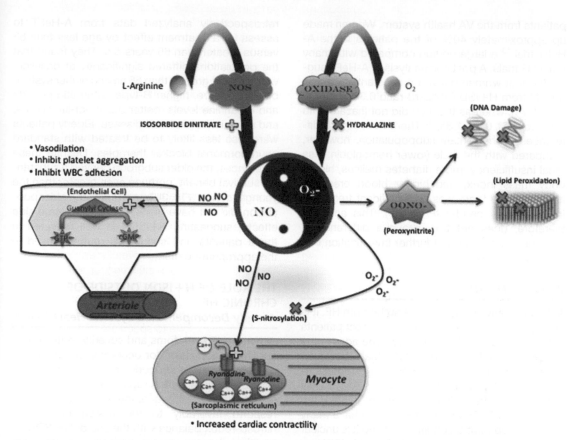

Fig. 2. The nitroso-redox balance. Maintaining a healthy balance between NO and ROS is vital to many fundamental processes in the human body. NO has far-reaching effects on the cardiovascular system through a variety of mechanisms, including up-regulation of intracellular cGMP via guanylyl cyclase activation, S-nitrosylation of effector proteins leading to downstream activation of the myocyte ryanodine receptor, and the formation of peroxynitrite, a toxic free radical with numerous deleterious effects. NOS, NO synthase. (*From* Cole RT, Kalogeropoulos AP, Georgiopoulou VV, et al. Hydralazine and isosorbide dinitrate in heart failure: historical perspective, mechanisms, and future directions. Circulation 2011;123(21):2414–22; with permission.)

study by Stein and colleagues[40] analyzing forearm blood flow responses to various agents, healthy black patients had an attenuated vasodilatory response to both methacholine (a stimulant of endothelium-dependent NO release) and nitroprusside (a stimulant of endothelium-independent NO release) compared with their white counterparts. Cardillo and colleagues[41] similarly showed that black patients had blunted vasodilatory responses to both acetylcholine and nitroprusside administration. A third study in a chronic HF population showed that black HF patients had greatly impaired endothelium-dependent, flow-mediated vasodilation.[42] Finally, blacks have been shown to produce greater levels of superoxide and, therefore, higher levels of peroxynitrite formation,[43] which has multiple deleterious cardiovascular effects, as discussed previously.

Considering these studies, it is feasible that black patients might derive a greater benefit from

the H+ISDN combination than their nonblack HF counterparts. Again, the absence of benefit in a large, nonblack HF population has never been proved in a study, such as A-HeFT, and these findings are merely hypothesis generating at best. Ultimately, the American College of Cardiology/American Heart Association guidelines give a class I recommendation for H+ISDN in all black HF patients with reduced EF and ongoing symptoms despite optimal medical therapy. For nonblacks, however, H+ISDN is given a IIA recommendation in addition to optimal medical therapy (and a IIB recommendation for those intolerant of ACEIs/angiotensin receptor blockers).[44]

Gender and H+ISDN

Of the 3 major clinical trials assessing the use of H+ISDN, only 1 (A-HeFT) included female patients. Both V-HeFT I and II enrolled only male patients from the VA health system. Women made up approximately 40% of the patients in the A-HeFT trial,[13] a large portion compared with many other HF trials. A post hoc analysis of A-HeFT suggested that women derived a substantial survival benefit from H+ISDN (hazard ratio 0.33; 95% CI, 0.16–0.71), whereas the men did not (hazard ratio 0.79; 95% CI, 0.46–1.35).[45] There were several differences in the female subpopulation, however, compared with the male (lower hemoglobin, less renal insufficiency, more diabetes mellitus, higher body mass index, and higher blood pressure) and ultimately there was no significant treatment interaction by gender (P = .47). This analysis, therefore, does not truly prove a difference in response by gender, but further investigation into this is warranted.

Age and H+ISDN

Although many young patients suffer from HF, it is largely a disease of the elderly, with most patients in their mid to late 70s.[46] The average ages in the V-HeFT I, V-HeFT II, and A-HeFT trials, however, were only 58, 60, and 57, respectively, representing relatively young HF populations.[9,10,13] Only 30% of the patients in A-HeFT were greater than 65 years old.[13] Older patients tend to have many significant comorbid conditions,[46] and it is unclear if they derive the same benefit from H+ISDN as their younger counterparts. Attempting to further address this question, Taylor and colleagues[47]

retrospectively analyzed data from A-HeFT to assess for a treatment effect by age less than 65 versus greater than 65 years old. They found that the populations differed significantly at baseline, with patients greater than 65 having higher systolic blood pressure, higher B-type natriuretic peptide and creatinine levels, better quality-of-life scores, and more ischemic heart disease. Elderly patients were also less likely to be treated with standard neurohormonal blocker therapies. Despite these differences, the older subgroup derived a substantial survival benefit, perhaps even greater than the younger cohort (**Fig. 3**). Importantly, the older population did not have higher rates of adverse side effects, suggesting H+ISDN is well tolerated in these patients and should be routinely used in the appropriate patients.

THE ROLE OF H+ISDN OUTSIDE OF CHRONIC HF
Acutely Decompensated Systolic Heart Failure

Although HF symptoms and severity exist along a spectrum, admission for decompensated HF is a sentinel event that forebodes poor outcomes.[48–50] Acute decompensation represents an extreme of oxidative stress,[51–53] and, therefore, patients may respond favorably to the restoration of the nitroso-redox balance with the use of H+ISDN. In addition, decompensation typically represents the extremes of hemodynamic perturbation (elevated preload and vascular resistance), and patients

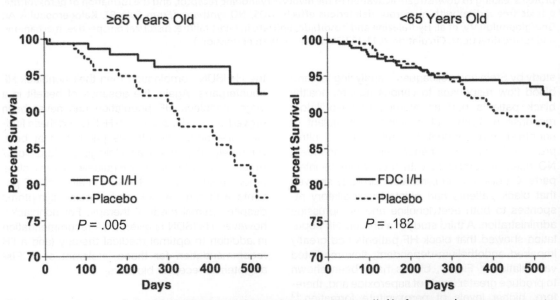

Fig. 3. Retrospective analysis of A-HeFT suggests that patients over 65 years (*left*) of age may have an even greater survival advantage with H+ISDN than patients less than 65 (*right*). FDC I/H, fixed-dose combination isosorbide/hydralazine. (*From* Taylor AL, Sabolinski ML, Tam SW, et al. Effect of fixed-dose combined isosorbide dinitrate/hydralazine in elderly patients in the African-American heart failure trial. J Card Fail 2012;18(8):600–6; with permission.)

may benefit from the preload- and afterload-reducing effects of these agents. Despite these hypotheses, there are few clinical data to assess the potential benefit of H+ISDN in acute decompensation. Mullens and colleagues[54] showed that H+ISDN can be useful when transitioning patients from intravenous nitroprusside to oral vasodilator therapy in the inpatient setting when patients present with low-output HF. Although this was not a randomized trial, such a strategy did lead to lower rates of all-cause mortality compared with a similar group of control patients (29% vs 44%; odds ratio 0.48; $P = .005$; 95% CI, 0.29–0.80), despite the vasodilator group having more deranged hemodynamics at baseline. Similarly, the in-hospital initiation of H+ISDN in addition to standard neurohormonal blockade was associated with improved outpatient survival in a study of 239 patients admitted with acute decompensation (34% vs 41%, odds ratio 0.65, 95% CI, 0.43 to 0.99; $P = .04$).[55] This survival benefit was found irrespective of race. This was not, however, a randomized placebo-controlled trial. Ultimately, further investigation is necessary to determine if H+ISDN is an effective therapy for the treatment of acutely decompensated HF.

Secondary Pulmonary Hypertension in Heart Failure

Many patients with HF have concomitant pulmonary hypertension, a process that can range from passive congestion to pulmonary vasoconstriction to irreversible anatomic changes in the pulmonary vascular bed.[56] The development of pulmonary hypertension in HF is associated with increased mortality[57–59] and can ultimately lead to right ventricular failure, also associated with poor outcomes.[60–63] NO plays a key role in the maintenance of vascular tone in the pulmonary bed as well as the vasodilatory response to endothelium-dependent stimuli.[64–66] Several experimental studies have revealed that HF is associated with impairments in NO-mediated pulmonary vasodilatation,[67–69] suggesting that the nitroso-redox balance may be as important in the pulmonary bed as it is in the systemic vasculature. It might, therefore, be speculated that pulmonary hypertension in HF could improve with H+ISDN therapy. Both Unverferth and colleagues[70] and Packer and colleagues[71] showed that the use of H+ISDN in HF patients improved pulmonary vascular resistance acutely and over the course of 3 months. These were small studies, however, and the effects of H+ISDN on pulmonary hypertension and right ventricular function have never been evaluated in a large-scale trial. This is an area that warrants further evaluation.

MAINTAINING THE NITROSO-REDOX BALANCE: IS HYDRALAZINE NECESSARY?
ACEIs + Nitrates

As previously discussed, the utility of H+ISDN in HF may result from its effects on the nitroso-redox balance, not the vasodilatory properties of the individual drugs. Although the role that ISDN plays in augmenting NO availability is clear, it has been postulated that alternative antioxidant agents might be substituted for hydralazine, obviating a thrice-a-day drug with many adverse side effects.[30] Most notable among these potential alternative agents are the ACEIs, which have antioxidant properties and inhibit the development of nitrate tolerance in both animal and human studies.[72–75] Clinically, the use of ACEIs as background therapy leads to more marked and sustained hemodynamic improvements when nitrates are added compared with nitrates alone.[73,74,76] In a small randomized controlled trial comparing transdermal nitroglycerin (NTG) with placebo in patients taking ACEIs at baseline, the NTG group showed significant improvements in left ventricular (LV) dimensions, LV fractional shortening, and exercise capacity,[33] suggesting this combination is safe and effective in HF patients. All of these studies of ACEIs and nitrate combinations, however, are small and hypothesis generating at best. There are also studies suggesting no benefit to combination therapy with ACEI and nitrates.[77–79] Nonetheless, this is an area that should be further investigated, because it could have a major impact on future pharmacotherapy in HF.

Other Agents + Nitrates

Other medications known to provide morbidity and mortality benefit in HF have also shown similar benefits when given in conjunction with chronic nitrate therapy. Carvedilol, unlike other β-blockers, decreases superoxide production and maintains vascular dilatation and even at small doses reduces nitrate tolerance.[80–84] Aldosterone antagonists have also been shown to decrease the oxidative stress that is associated with elevated circulating aldosterone levels in HF,[85–88] although no large-scale studies to date have specifically addressed these effects on nitrate tolerance and the nitroso-redox balance. In light of these findings, again the true utility of hydralazine when used in combination with nitrates in patients already on background therapy with ACEIs, carvedilol, and aldosterone antagonists may be speculated on, warranting ongoing investigation.

H+ISDN IN CLINICAL PRACTICE

Despite the well-documented clinical benefits of H+ISDN and the substantial mortality improvement in black HF patients, the use of this combination is low in clinical practice. A prospective analysis of treatment trends in more than 15,000 patients from the IMPROVE-HF cohort revealed that only 7% of eligible black HF patients receive H+ISDN (**Fig. 4**).[89] Similarly, in a large registry of hospitalized HF patients, less than 5% of black patients were discharged on H+ISDN.[90] Finally, a recent analysis of more than 54,000 patients admitted with decompensated HF (Get With the Guidelines registry) revealed that only 12.6% of the patients eligible for H+ISDN received these agents.[91] The rates of H+ISDN in African American patients improve to 24% by the end of the study, but this is inadequate when considering the potential magnitude of benefit in this population.

The reasons for low prescription rates for H+ISDN are manifold. The thrice-daily dosing creates difficulties with patient compliance and may result in underdosing by both patients and providers. Side effects with these agents at the recommended doses are common as well, including headaches (47.5%) and dizziness (29.3%).[13] This can lead to dose reductions to potentially subtherapeutic levels and may affect patient compliance. Many male patients with HF suffer from concomitant erectile dysfunction related to medical comorbidities and β-blocker use. Thus, they frequently use type 5 phosphodiesterase inhibitors (eg, sildenafil, tadalafil, and vardenafil), which are contraindicated in patients taking nitrate therapies. Finally, the costs associated with the BiDil formulation used in the clinical trial are often an important consideration when prescribing H+ISDN. Although it is common in clinical practice to simply substitute the individual components of BiDil with generic equivalents, there are data to suggest alternative formulations may not achieve the same therapeutic levels as the BiDil product.[92]

Ultimately, it is clear that utilization of H+ISDN in HF patients is poor. Ongoing efforts to educate both patients and physicians on the major benefits

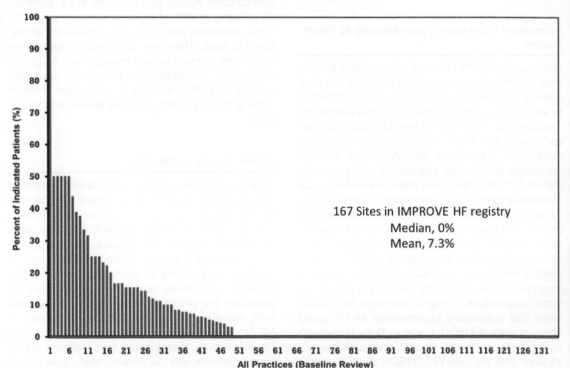

Fig. 4. Despite the well-documented clinical benefits of H+ISDN in black HF patients, the use of this combination is low in clinical practice. Data from a prospective analysis of treatment trends in more than 15,000 patients in the IMPROVE-HF cohort revealed that only 7% of eligible black HF patients receive H+ISDN. HYD, hydralazine. (*From* Yancy CW, Fonarow GC, Albert NM, et al. Adherence to guideline-recommended adjunctive heart failure therapies among outpatient cardiology practices [findings from IMPROVE HF]. Am J Cardiol 2010;105(2):255–60; with permission.)

of these drugs must continue to achieve better outcomes, particularly in the black HF population.

SUMMARY

The modern history of HF pharmacotherapy parallels the history of H+ISDN, beginning with the first ever large-scale, randomized controlled trial in HF: V-HeFT I. Initially used for the balanced vasodilatory properties of each drug and its individual effects on preload/afterload, it is now known there is more to the story. In truth, the maintenance of the nitroso-redox balance may be the true underlying mechanism of benefit of these drugs.

Since the publication of V-HeFT I approximately 30 years ago, H+ISDN has been the subject of much discussion and debate. Although the benefits of this therapy seem clear in black HF patients, its utility in other populations has never been studied on a similar scale (and likely never will be); therefore, there will continue to be ongoing doubts about the use of H+ISDN in nonblack HF patients. Substudies of the A-HeFT trial have also suggested that there may or may not be preferential benefit in specific subsets of patients, including women with HF and the elderly. Ongoing investigation is necessary, however, to fully understand these hypothesis-generating results.

Finally, there is evidence to suggest that other commonly used HF medications (ACEIs, carvedilol, and aldosterone antagonists) may be as effective as hydralazine at reducing the effects of oxidative stress and the development of nitrate tolerance. This is an area that warrants further investigation in light of the many issues associated with hydralazine use.

Regardless of the many controversies surrounding H+ISDN, one thing is clear: this therapy is grossly underutilized in clinical practice and many patients who could benefit from H+ISDN never receive the drugs. Ongoing physician and patient education is mandatory to improve the rates of H+ISDN use.

REFERENCES

1. Cohn JN, Franciosa JA. Vasodilator therapy of cardiac failure (second of two parts). N Engl J Med 1977;297(5):254–8.
2. Bertel O, Steiner A. Rotating tourniquets do not work in acute congestive heart failure and pulmonary oedema. Lancet 1980;1(8171):762.
3. Cohn JN. Vasodilator therapy for heart failure. The influence of impedance on left ventricular performance. Circulation 1973;48(1):5–8.
4. Cole RT, Kalogeropoulos AP, Georgiopoulou VV, et al. Hydralazine and isosorbide dinitrate in heart failure: historical perspective, mechanisms, and future directions. Circulation 2011;123(21):2414–22.
5. Franciosa JA, Limas CJ, Guiha NH, et al. Improved left ventricular function during nitroprusside infusion in acute myocardial infarction. Lancet 1972; 1(7752):650–4.
6. Guiha NH, Cohn JN, Mikulic E, et al. Treatment of refractory heart failure with infusion of nitroprusside. N Engl J Med 1974;291(12):587–92.
7. Massie B, Chatterjee K, Werner J, et al. Hemodynamic advantage of combined administration of hydralazine orally and nitrates nonparenterally in the vasodilator therapy of chronic heart failure. Am J Cardiol 1977;40(5):794–801.
8. Pierpont GL, Cohn JN, Franciosa JA. Combined oral hydralazine-nitrate therapy in left ventricular failure. Hemodynamic equivalency to sodium nitroprusside. Chest 1978;73(1):8–13.
9. Cohn JN, Archibald DG, Ziesche S, et al. Effect of vasodilator therapy on mortality in chronic congestive heart failure. Results of a Veterans Administration Cooperative Study. N Engl J Med 1986; 314(24):1547–52.
10. Cohn JN, Johnson G, Ziesche S, et al. A comparison of enalapril with hydralazine-isosorbide dinitrate in the treatment of chronic congestive heart failure. N Engl J Med 1991;325(5):303–10.
11. Effects of enalapril on mortality in severe congestive heart failure. Results of the Cooperative North Scandinavian Enalapril Survival Study (CONSENSUS). The CONSENSUS Trial Study Group. N Engl J Med 1987;316(23):1429–35.
12. Carson P, Ziesche S, Johnson G, et al. Racial differences in response to therapy for heart failure: analysis of the vasodilator-heart failure trials. Vasodilator-Heart Failure Trial Study Group. J Card Fail 1999; 5(3):178–87.
13. Taylor AL, Ziesche S, Yancy C, et al. Combination of isosorbide dinitrate and hydralazine in blacks with heart failure. N Engl J Med 2004;351(20): 2049–57.
14. O'Connor CM, Starling RC, Hernandez AF, et al. Effect of nesiritide in patients with acute decompensated heart failure. N Engl J Med 2011;365(1):32–43.
15. Cuffe MS, Califf RM, Adams KF Jr, et al. Short-term intravenous milrinone for acute exacerbation of chronic heart failure: a randomized controlled trial. JAMA 2002;287(12):1541–7.
16. Packer M, O'Connor CM, Ghali JK, et al. Effect of amlodipine on morbidity and mortality in severe chronic heart failure. Prospective Randomized Amlodipine Survival Evaluation Study Group. N Engl J Med 1996;335(15):1107–14.
17. Packer M, McMurray J, Massie BM, et al. Clinical effects of endothelin receptor antagonism with bosentan in patients with severe chronic heart failure: results of a pilot study. J Card Fail 2005;11(1):12–20.

18. Cole RT, Gheorghiade M, Georgiopoulou VV, et al. Reassessing the use of vasodilators in heart failure. Expert Rev Cardiovasc Ther 2012;10(9):1141–51.

19. Hare JM. Nitroso-redox balance in the cardiovascular system. N Engl J Med 2004;351(20):2112–4.

20. Keith M, Geranmayegan A, Sole MJ, et al. Increased oxidative stress in patients with congestive heart failure. J Am Coll Cardiol 1998;31(6):1352–6.

21. McMurray J, Chopra M, Abdullah I, et al. Evidence of oxidative stress in chronic heart failure in humans. Eur Heart J 1993;14(11):1493–8.

22. Yucel D, Aydogdu S, Cehreli S, et al. Increased oxidative stress in dilated cardiomyopathic heart failure. Clin Chem 1998;44(1):148–54.

23. Wink DA, Mitchell JB. Chemical biology of nitric oxide: insights into regulatory, cytotoxic, and cytoprotective mechanisms of nitric oxide. Free Radic Biol Med 1998;25(4–5):434–56.

24. Stamler JS, Lamas S, Fang FC. Nitrosylation. The prototypic redox-based signaling mechanism. Cell 2001;106(6):675–83.

25. Xu L, Eu JP, Meissner G, et al. Activation of the cardiac calcium release channel (ryanodine receptor) by poly-S-nitrosylation. Science 1998;279(5348):234–7.

26. Gonzalez DR, Treuer AV, Castellanos J, et al. Impaired S-nitrosylation of the ryanodine receptor caused by xanthine oxidase activity contributes to calcium leak in heart failure. J Biol Chem 2010;285(37):28938–45.

27. Arstall MA, Sawyer DB, Fukazawa R, et al. Cytokine-mediated apoptosis in cardiac myocytes: the role of inducible nitric oxide synthase induction and peroxynitrite generation. Circ Res 1999;85(9):829–40.

28. Levrand S, Vannay-Bouchiche C, Pesse B, et al. Peroxynitrite is a major trigger of cardiomyocyte apoptosis in vitro and in vivo. Free Radic Biol Med 2006;41(6):886–95.

29. Pacher P, Beckman JS, Liaudet L. Nitric oxide and peroxynitrite in health and disease. Physiol Rev 2007;87(1):315–424.

30. Gupta D, Georgiopoulou VV, Kalogeropoulos AP, et al. Nitrate therapy for heart failure: benefits and strategies to overcome tolerance. JACC Heart Fail 2013;1(3):183–91.

31. Foster MW, McMahon TJ, Stamler JS. S-nitrosylation in health and disease. Trends Mol Med 2003;9(4):160–8.

32. Viner RI, Williams TD, Schoneich C. Nitric oxide-dependent modification of the sarcoplasmic reticulum Ca-ATPase: localization of cysteine target sites. Free Radic Biol Med 2000;29(6):489–96.

33. Elkayam U, Johnson JV, Shotan A, et al. Double-blind, placebo-controlled study to evaluate the effect of organic nitrates in patients with chronic heart failure treated with angiotensin-converting enzyme inhibition. Circulation 1999;99(20):2652–7.

34. Leiro JM, Alvarez E, Arranz JA, et al. Antioxidant activity and inhibitory effects of hydralazine on inducible NOS/COX-2 gene and protein expression in rat peritoneal macrophages. Int Immunopharmacol 2004;4(2):163–77.

35. Daiber A, Oelze M, Coldewey M, et al. Hydralazine is a powerful inhibitor of peroxynitrite formation as a possible explanation for its beneficial effects on prognosis in patients with congestive heart failure. Biochem Biophys Res Commun 2005;338(4):1865–74.

36. Daiber A, Mulsch A, Hink U, et al. The oxidative stress concept of nitrate tolerance and the antioxidant properties of hydralazine. Am J Cardiol 2005;96(7B):25i–36i.

37. Munzel T, Kurz S, Rajagopalan S, et al. Hydralazine prevents nitroglycerin tolerance by inhibiting activation of a membrane-bound NADH oxidase. A new action for an old drug. J Clin Invest 1996;98(6):1465–70.

38. Gogia H, Mehra A, Parikh S, et al. Prevention of tolerance to hemodynamic effects of nitrates with concomitant use of hydralazine in patients with chronic heart failure. J Am Coll Cardiol 1995;26(7):1575–80.

39. Dulce RA, Yiginer O, Gonzalez DR, et al. Hydralazine and organic nitrates restore impaired excitation-contraction coupling by reducing calcium leak associated with nitroso-redox imbalance. J Biol Chem 2013;288(9):6522–33.

40. Stein CM, Lang CC, Nelson R, et al. Vasodilation in black Americans: attenuated nitric oxide-mediated responses. Clin Pharmacol Ther 1997;62(4):436–43.

41. Cardillo C, Kilcoyne CM, Cannon RO 3rd, et al. Attenuation of cyclic nucleotide-mediated smooth muscle relaxation in blacks as a cause of racial differences in vasodilator function. Circulation 1999;99(1):90–5.

42. Androne AS, Hryniewicz K, Hudaihed A, et al. Comparison of metabolic vasodilation in response to exercise and ischemia and endothelium-dependent flow-mediated dilation in African-American versus non-African-American patients with chronic heart failure. Am J Cardiol 2006;97(5):685–9.

43. Kalinowski L, Dobrucki IT, Malinski T. Race-specific differences in endothelial function: predisposition of African Americans to vascular diseases. Circulation 2004;109(21):2511–7.

44. Hunt SA, Abraham WT, Chin MH, et al. 2009 focused update incorporated into the ACC/AHA 2005 Guidelines for the Diagnosis and Management of Heart Failure in Adults: a report of the American College of Cardiology Foundation/American Heart Association Task Force on Practice Guidelines: developed in collaboration with the

International Society for Heart and Lung Transplantation. Circulation 2009;119(14):e391–479.

45. Taylor AL, Lindenfeld J, Ziesche S, et al. Outcomes by gender in the African-American Heart Failure Trial. J Am Coll Cardiol 2006;48(11):2263–7.

46. Mosterd A, Hoes AW. Clinical epidemiology of heart failure. Heart 2007;93(9):1137–46.

47. Taylor AL, Sabolinski ML, Tam SW, et al. Effect of fixed-dose combined isosorbide dinitrate/hydralazine in elderly patients in the African-American heart failure trial. J Card Fail 2012;18(8):600–6.

48. Fonarow GC, Adams KF Jr, Abraham WT, et al. Risk stratification for in-hospital mortality in acutely decompensated heart failure: classification and regression tree analysis. JAMA 2005; 293(5):572–80.

49. Ross JS, Chen J, Lin Z, et al. Recent national trends in readmission rates after heart failure hospitalization. Circ Heart Fail 2010;3(1):97–103.

50. Shahar E, Lee S, Kim J, et al. Hospitalized heart failure: rates and long-term mortality. J Card Fail 2004;10(5):374–9.

51. Hokamaki J, Kawano H, Yoshimura M, et al. Urinary biopyrrins levels are elevated in relation to severity of heart failure. J Am Coll Cardiol 2004;43(10): 1880–5.

52. Testa M, Yeh M, Lee P, et al. Circulating levels of cytokines and their endogenous modulators in patients with mild to severe congestive heart failure due to coronary artery disease or hypertension. J Am Coll Cardiol 1996;28(4):964–71.

53. Ungvari Z, Gupte SA, Recchia FA, et al. Role of oxidative-nitrosative stress and downstream pathways in various forms of cardiomyopathy and heart failure. Curr Vasc Pharmacol 2005;3(3):221–9.

54. Mullens W, Abrahams Z, Francis GS, et al. Sodium nitroprusside for advanced low-output heart failure. J Am Coll Cardiol 2008;52(3):200–7.

55. Mullens W, Abrahams Z, Francis GS, et al. Usefulness of Isosorbide dinitrate and hydralazine as add-on therapy in patients discharged for advanced decompensated heart failure. Am J Cardiol 2009; 103(8):1113–9.

56. Guazzi M, Borlaug BA. Pulmonary hypertension due to left heart disease. Circulation 2012;126(8): 975–90.

57. Ghio S, Gavazzi A, Campana C, et al. Independent and additive prognostic value of right ventricular systolic function and pulmonary artery pressure in patients with chronic heart failure. J Am Coll Cardiol 2001;37(1):183–8.

58. Abramson SV, Burke JF, Kelly JJ Jr, et al. Pulmonary hypertension predicts mortality and morbidity in patients with dilated cardiomyopathy. Ann Intern Med 1992;116(11):888–95.

59. Kjaergaard J, Akkan D, Iversen KK, et al. Prognostic importance of pulmonary hypertension in

patients with heart failure. Am J Cardiol 2007; 99(8):1146–50.

60. de Groote P, Millaire A, Foucher-Hossein C, et al. Right ventricular ejection fraction is an independent predictor of survival in patients with moderate heart failure. J Am Coll Cardiol 1998;32(4):948–54.

61. Di Salvo TG, Mathier M, Semigran MJ, et al. Preserved right ventricular ejection fraction predicts exercise capacity and survival in advanced heart failure. J Am Coll Cardiol 1995;25(5):1143–53.

62. Field ME, Solomon SD, Lewis EF, et al. Right ventricular dysfunction and adverse outcome in patients with advanced heart failure. J Card Fail 2006;12(8):616–20.

63. Juilliere Y, Barbier G, Feldmann L, et al. Additional predictive value of both left and right ventricular ejection fractions on long-term survival in idiopathic dilated cardiomyopathy. Eur Heart J 1997;18(2): 276–80.

64. Blitzer ML, Loh E, Roddy MA, et al. Endothelium-derived nitric oxide regulates systemic and pulmonary vascular resistance during acute hypoxia in humans. J Am Coll Cardiol 1996;28(3):591–6.

65. Cooper CJ, Landzberg MJ, Anderson TJ, et al. Role of nitric oxide in the local regulation of pulmonary vascular resistance in humans. Circulation 1996;93(2):266–71.

66. Stamler JS, Loh E, Roddy MA, et al. Nitric oxide regulates basal systemic and pulmonary vascular resistance in healthy humans. Circulation 1994; 89(5):2035–40.

67. Ontkean M, Gay R, Greenberg B. Diminished endothelium-derived relaxing factor activity in an experimental model of chronic heart failure. Circ Res 1991;69(4):1088–96.

68. Porter TR, Taylor DO, Cycan A, et al. Endothelium-dependent pulmonary artery responses in chronic heart failure: influence of pulmonary hypertension. J Am Coll Cardiol 1993;22(5):1418–24.

69. Cooper CJ, Jevnikar FW, Walsh T, et al. The influence of basal nitric oxide activity on pulmonary vascular resistance in patients with congestive heart failure. Am J Cardiol 1998;82(5):609–14.

70. Unverferth DV, Mehegan JP, Magorien RD, et al. Regression of myocardial cellular hypertrophy with vasodilator therapy in chronic congestive heart failure associated with idiopathic dilated cardiomyopathy. Am J Cardiol 1983;51(8):1392–8.

71. Packer M, Medina N, Yushak M. Contrasting hemodynamic responses in severe heart failure: comparison of captopril and other vasodilator drugs. Am Heart J 1982;104(5 Pt 2):1215–23.

72. Kurz S, Hink U, Nickenig G, et al. Evidence for a causal role of the renin-angiotensin system in nitrate tolerance. Circulation 1999;99(24):3181–7.

73. Mehra A, Ostrzega E, Shotan A, et al. Persistent hemodynamic improvement with short-term nitrate

therapy in patients with chronic congestive heart failure already treated with captopril. Am J Cardiol 1992;70(15):1310–4.

74. Stork T, Eichstadt H, Mockel M, et al. Hemodynamic action of captopril in coronary patients with heart failure tolerant to nitroglycerin. Clin Cardiol 1997;20(12):999–1004.

75. Katz RJ, Levy WS, Buff L, et al. Prevention of nitrate tolerance with angiotension converting enzyme inhibitors. Circulation 1991;83(4):1271–7.

76. Pizzulli L, Hagendorff A, Zirbes M, et al. Influence of captopril on nitroglycerin-mediated vasodilation and development of nitrate tolerance in arterial and venous circulation. Am Heart J 1996;131(2):342–9.

77. Dakak N, Makhoul N, Flugelman MY, et al. Failure of captopril to prevent nitrate tolerance in congestive heart failure secondary to coronary artery disease. Am J Cardiol 1990;66(5):608–13.

78. Dupuis J, Lalonde G, Bichet D, et al. Captopril does not prevent nitroglycerin tolerance in heart failure. Can J Cardiol 1990;6(7):281–6.

79. Parker JD, Parker JO. Effect of therapy with an angiotensin-converting enzyme inhibitor on hemodynamic and counterregulatory responses during continuous therapy with nitroglycerin. J Am Coll Cardiol 1993;21(6):1445–53.

80. El-Demerdash E. Evidences for prevention of nitroglycerin tolerance by carvedilol. Pharm Res 2006; 53(4):380–5.

81. Fink B, Schwemmer M, Fink N, et al. Tolerance to nitrates with enhanced radical formation suppressed by carvedilol. J Cardiovasc Pharmacol 1999;34(6):800–5.

82. Nakahira A, Minamiyama Y, Takemura S, et al. Coadministration of carvedilol attenuates nitrate tolerance by preventing cytochrome p450 depletion. Circ J 2010;74(8):1711–7.

83. Watanabe H, Kakihana M, Ohtsuka S, et al. Preventive effects of carvedilol on nitrate tolerance–a randomized, double-blind, placebo-controlled comparative study between carvedilol and arotinolol. J Am Coll Cardiol 1998;32(5):1201–6.

84. Watanabe H, Kakihana M, Ohtsuka S, et al. Randomized, double-blind, placebo-controlled study of carvedilol on the prevention of nitrate tolerance in patients with chronic heart failure. J Am Coll Cardiol 1998;32(5):1194–200.

85. Pitt B. Effect of aldosterone blockade in patients with systolic left ventricular dysfunction: implications of the RALES and EPHESUS studies. Mol Cell Endocrinol 2004;217(1–2):53–8.

86. Sun Y, Zhang J, Lu L, et al. Aldosterone-induced inflammation in the rat heart: role of oxidative stress. Am J Pathol 2002;161(5):1773–81.

87. Toda N, Nakanishi S, Tanabe S. Aldosterone affects blood flow and vascular tone regulated by endothelium-derived NO: therapeutic implications. Br J Pharmacol 2013;168(3):519–33.

88. Skott O, Uhrenholt TR, Schjerning J, et al. Rapid actions of aldosterone in vascular health and disease–friend or foe? Pharmacol Ther 2006;111(2): 495–507.

89. Yancy CW, Fonarow GC, Albert NM, et al. Adherence to guideline-recommended adjunctive heart failure therapies among outpatient cardiology practices (findings from IMPROVE HF). Am J Cardiol 2010;105(2):255–60.

90. Yancy CW, Abraham WT, Albert NM, et al. Quality of care of and outcomes for African Americans hospitalized with heart failure: findings from the OPTIMIZE-HF (Organized Program to Initiate Lifesaving Treatment in Hospitalized Patients With Heart Failure) registry. J Am Coll Cardiol 2008;51(17):1675–84.

91. Golwala HB, Thadani U, Liang L, et al. Use of hydralazine-isosorbide dinitrate combination in African American and other race/ethnic group patients with heart failure and reduced left ventricular ejection fraction. J Am Heart Assoc 2013;2(4):e000214.

92. Tam SW, Sabolinski ML, Worcel M, et al. Lack of bioequivalence between different formulations of isosorbide dinitrate and hydralazine and the fixed-dose combination of isosorbide dinitrate/hydralazine: the V-HeFT paradox. Clin Pharm 2007; 46(10):885–95.

Polypharmacy in Heart Failure: Drugs to Use and Avoid

Brent N. Reed, PharmD[a], Jo E. Rodgers, PharmD[b], Carla A. Sueta, MD, PhD[c],*

KEYWORDS

• Heart failure • Comorbidities • Polypharmacy

KEY POINTS

• Polypharmacy due to combination medication regimens for the management of heart failure (HF), treatment of comorbidities, and high use of nonprescription drugs is universal.
• Therapeutic dilemmas, including drug-disease interactions and drug-drug interactions between both prescription and nonprescription medications are common.
• Careful evaluation and monitoring of potentially deleterious effects that may result from multidrug regimens is strongly recommended.

INTRODUCTION

Polypharmacy, the use of 4 or more drugs, in patients with heart failure (HF) is universal. Patients with HF with reduced ejection fraction (HFrEF) are prescribed combination therapy, including a diuretic, angiotensin-converting enzyme inhibitor (ACEI) or angiotensin receptor blocker (ARB), beta-blocker (BB), aldosterone receptor antagonist (ARA), and digoxin, as endorsed by practice guidelines.[1] Management of common comorbidities and use of nonprescription therapies add to the complexity of medication regimens in patients with HF, which may impact adherence and increase the risk of adverse drug reactions, and drug-disease or drug-drug interactions. Included in this review are strategies for optimizing combination therapy used to manage HFrEF and common comorbidities, as well as medications to avoid or use with caution.

EVIDENCE-BASED COMBINATION THERAPY IN HEART FAILURE WITH REDUCED EJECTION FRACTION
Determination of Volume Status

Many factors impact volume status, including salt and fluid intake, progression of disease, declining renal function, and treatment of comorbidities. Loop diuretics (eg, furosemide, bumetanide, torsemide) are most often used to maintain euvolemia. For patients requiring diuretic therapy, the lowest effective dose is recommended, as diuretics stimulate compensatory neurohormonal systems and may lead to disease progression. Dose escalation is often required to maintain euvolemia as HF progresses. If twice-daily dosing is required, the second dose should be administered in the afternoon to minimize nocturia. Furosemide is the most commonly used loop diuretic, but bumetanide and torsemide may be considered in patients failing to respond to furosemide due to improved bioavailability. Alternatively, the addition of a thiazidelike diuretic (eg, hydrochlorothiazide, chlorothiazide, metolazone) may be considered to augment diuresis. Thiazidelike diuretics possess mild vasodilatory properties, which may decrease blood pressure, and with the exception of metolazone, are generally less effective in patients with advanced renal impairment (ie, glomerular filtration rate [GFR] less than 30 mL/min). Electrolytes should be carefully monitored, as combination diuretic therapy may result in significant electrolyte abnormalities, hypovolemia, and acute kidney

Disclosures: None.
[a] Department of Pharmacy Practice and Science, University of Maryland School of Pharmacy, Baltimore, MD, USA; [b] Division of Pharmacotherapy and Experimental Therapeutics, University of North Carolina Eshelman School of Pharmacy, Chapel Hill, NC, USA; [c] UNC Center for Heart and Vascular Care, University of North Carolina at Chapel Hill, 160 Dental Circle, Chapel Hill, NC 27599, USA
* Corresponding author.
E-mail address: carla_sueta@med.unc.edu

Heart Failure Clin 10 (2014) 577–590
http://dx.doi.org/10.1016/j.hfc.2014.07.005
1551-7136/14/$ – see front matter © 2014 Elsevier Inc. All rights reserved.

injury. Adding an ARA to a loop diuretic may also augment diuresis but should be avoided in patients with GFR less than 30 mL/min or a serum potassium greater than 5.0 mEq/L.

In the setting of hypovolemia, diuretics should be decreased or discontinued and oral hydration (or in severe cases, careful infusion of intravenous fluids) should be administered. Other evidence-based therapy (ACEI/ARB, ARA) should not be added in hypovolemic patients, as hypotension, ongoing diuresis, and/or acute kidney injury may result.

Addition of ACE Inhibitor or Angiotensin Receptor Blocker

ACEIs and ARBs reduce mortality and HF hospitalizations in patients with symptomatic HFrEF.[1] However, ARBs are not superior to ACEIs and should generally be reserved for those with a history of ACEI intolerance (ie, cough, angioedema).[2,3] If patients develop cough, alternative etiologies should be considered (eg, volume overload, lung disease) before changing to an ARB. Both therapies are associated with similar rates of renal impairment, hyperkalemia, and hypotension, but are generally well tolerated when initiated in euvolemic patients or in combination with a diuretic in patients who are hypervolemic. Initial doses depend on blood pressure and can be increased every 1 to 2 weeks (or every 1–2 days in hospitalized patients) as tolerated, as up-titration to target doses results in additional decreases in HF hospitalizations.[4,5] An increase in serum creatinine should be expected after initiation of therapy, and renal function should be monitored at baseline and 1 to 2 weeks after initiation of therapy. If renal function significantly worsens, bilateral renal artery stenosis should be suspected and therapy discontinued. Serum potassium also should be monitored at baseline and 1 to 2 weeks after initiation of therapy, although concentrations less than 5.5 mEq/L are acceptable.

Addition of BB

Addition of a BB to ACEI or ARB therapy further reduces mortality across the spectrum of chronic HFrEF, as well as all-cause hospitalizations and HF hospitalizations.[1] Dose-related reverse remodeling and improvement in left ventricular ejection fraction (LVEF) are also observed, with the most significant gains occurring in those with hypertensive or idiopathic cardiomyopathies.[6] Because of these benefits, we recommend adding a BB to ACEI or ARB therapy early (ie, before complete up-titration of ACEI/ARB to target dose).

Bisoprolol, carvedilol, and metoprolol succinate are preferred based on evidence from randomized controlled trials.[7-9] Selection of a specific BB is often influenced by a patient's comorbidities (additional details provided later in this article). Carvedilol is often selected for patients with hypertension, although its alpha-mediated vasodilating effects may diminish with chronic use.[10] The β_1-selective agents, bisoprolol and metoprolol succinate, are better tolerated in patients with lower blood pressure but have a greater impact on heart rate. Initiation or up-titration of BB therapy should be delayed in patients with evidence of volume overload (ie, presence of rales and more than minimal edema) to avoid decompensation. Once patients are euvolemic, therapy may be initiated safely before discharge. Initial doses are low because of a potential negative inotropic effect, but can usually be doubled every 2 weeks until the target or maximally tolerated dose is achieved, as dose-related improvements have been demonstrated with all 3 agents.[6,11,12] Assessment for adverse effects (eg, hypotension, bradycardia) and signs or symptoms of worsening HF (eg, fatigue, fluid overload) should be performed before dose titration. If decompensation occurs, diuretic dose may be increased, or the dose of BB may be decreased temporarily, but abrupt discontinuation should be avoided in the absence of overt cardiogenic shock. Fatigue and fluid retention are common adverse effects. Fatigue may be minimized by lengthening the time between dose titration, increasing doses by smaller increments, taking once-daily therapies at night, or switching to another BB. Fluid retention may be minimized by patient self-monitoring of daily weight with instructions for diuretic titration or when to contact a provider. If patients do not tolerate a BB or dose up-titration, referral to an HF specialist is recommended.

Addition of ARA and/or Nitrates Plus Hydralazine

Addition of an ARA (eplerenone or spironolactone) to ACEI or ARB plus BB therapy further improves all-cause mortality and reduces hospitalizations (including HF hospitalizations) in patients with New York Heart Association (NYHA) Class II to IV HFrEF.[13,14] Use of an ARA also improves ventricular function and HF symptoms regardless of baseline LVEF or NYHA class.[15] ARAs are recommended in patients with symptomatic HFrEF who have a serum creatinine less than 2.5 mg/dL or GFR greater than 30 mL/min/1.73 m^2 and serum potassium less than 5.0 mEq/L.[1] Initiation should be avoided in hypovolemic patients, as ARAs may augment diuresis, especially at higher doses. Aldosterone antagonists are usually initiated at 25 mg daily; although lower doses or alternate day dosing may be considered in patients with renal impairment or diabetes due to an increased risk of hyperkalemia. Serum potassium concentrations should not exceed 5.5 mEq/dL, and potassium supplementation (including use of potassium-containing salt substitutes) should be reduced or discontinued. Serum potassium and serum creatinine should be monitored at baseline, within 1 week, and monthly for at least the first 3 months after initiation. Eplerenone possesses less androgenic activity compared with spironolactone, thereby minimizing the risk of gynecomastia.

The combination of nitrates and hydralazine also prolongs survival, reduces hospitalizations (including HF hospitalizations), and improves symptoms in African Americans with NYHA class III to IV HF who are already receiving ACEI or ARB plus BB therapy.[16] It also may be considered as an alternative in patients with intolerance to ACEI or ARB (eg, renal insufficiency, hypotension, allergies).[1] Initial doses depend on baseline blood pressure, but those with low blood pressure derive similar benefit when compared with normotensive patients.[17] Dizziness and headache are the most common adverse effects but can be minimized by initiating therapy at low doses. Phosphodiesterase-5 inhibitors (eg, sildenafil) should not be prescribed with nitrates because of risks of hypotension.

Additional Pharmacologic Therapies for Heart Failure with Reduced Ejection Fraction

Digoxin reduces hospitalizations and improves symptoms and exercise tolerance but does not prolong survival in patients with HFrEF.[18] Because BB therapy is generally more effective at controlling ventricular rate, we generally recommend the addition of digoxin only after maximally tolerated doses of a BB have been achieved, although earlier use may be considered in patients with severe symptoms. A serum concentration of 0.5 to 0.9 ng/mL (<1 ng/mL) should be targeted, as benefits are observed at low serum concentrations and higher concentrations are associated with increased mortality, especially among women.[19] A common maintenance dose is 0.125 µg daily, but adjustments should be considered in patients with renal impairment, advanced age, low body mass, and in the presence of drug-drug interactions (eg, amiodarone). Digoxin toxicity may precipitate arrhythmias, and cause gastrointestinal and neurologic complaints.

Finally, omega-3 polyunsaturated fatty acids may be added to optimal medical therapy, as they improve mortality, LVEF, exercise tolerance, and symptoms.[20,21]

Combination Renin-Angiotensin-Aldosterone System Blockade

The combination of an ACEI and an ARB has been shown to reduce cardiovascular death and HF hospitalizations in patients with chronic HFrEF, although a recent meta-analysis reported no benefit compared with monotherapy in terms of total mortality and cardiovascular mortality.[22,23] The combination may be considered in patients with intolerance to BB, but should not be used in combination with an ARA because of an increased risk of hyperkalemia, renal dysfunction, and hypotension.

Renin Inhibitors

Addition of the direct renin inhibitor aliskiren to standard therapy does not improve HF outcomes and increases the risk of renal failure and hypotension.[24] In patients without diabetes, aliskiren is generally well-tolerated and may improve survival at 12 months, whereas mortality increases in those with diabetes. Based on the evidence to date, its use is not recommended in patients with HF.

PHARMACOLOGIC MANAGEMENT OF COMMON COMORBIDITIES

The presence of 5 or more comorbidities has been observed in up to 58% of patients with HF.[25,26] Risk of hospitalization increases with the number of comorbidities and several are associated with increased mortality and HF hospitalizations.[26] The pharmacologic management of these comorbidities often presents therapeutic dilemmas, such as drug-disease and drug-drug interactions, adverse drug events, and reduced compliance. Simplification of medication regimens, coordination of care, and multidisciplinary involvement are therefore paramount to the management of this patient population.

Conditions Requiring Use of Antiplatelet and Anticoagulant Therapy

Evidence for a benefit of aspirin in the absence of atherosclerotic disease is lacking, as it has not been shown to reduce cardiovascular events in patients with HF and normal sinus rhythm.[27–29] A meta-analysis of primary prevention trials found that although aspirin decreased nonfatal vascular events, a net benefit was not observed because of increased bleeding.[30] Current evidence is insufficient to recommend aspirin for primary prevention in patients with HF who are free of atherosclerotic disease and do not have compelling risk factors. Its use should be reserved for secondary prevention of conditions in which it has known benefits (eg, previous myocardial infarction or stroke). Given absence of a dose-related effect, 81 to 100 mg per day is recommended.

Addition of a P2Y12 inhibitor (ie, dual antiplatelet therapy) occurs in patients with a recent ischemic event and/or percutaneous coronary intervention. Clopidogrel is the most widely used agent in this class, but the more potent P2Y12 inhibitors prasugrel and ticagrelor have been associated with a greater reduction in cardiovascular events.[31,32] Compared with clopidogrel, prasugrel increases bleeding, whereas bleeding risk with ticagrelor is similar. Few patients with HF have been enrolled in trials of prasugrel or ticagrelor.

Anticoagulant therapy is recommended for patients with thromboembolic disease or those with atrial fibrillation and excess risk of stroke or systemic embolism (ie, CHA_2DS_2-VASc score ≥ 2). In trials of patients with HF and normal sinus rhythm, reductions in stroke are offset by increases in excess bleeding.[27–29] Warfarin has been the mainstay of anticoagulation therapy in HF, but is characterized by wide interpatient variability, especially in advanced disease. Newer oral anticoagulants, including apixaban, dabigatran, and rivaroxaban, have not been studied exclusively in HF, although significant numbers of patients with HF were enrolled in landmark trials: approximately 35%, 32%, and 62% of patients in trials of apixaban, dabigatran, and rivaroxaban, respectively.[33–35] A comparison of these agents can be found in **Table 1**. How the newer oral anticoagulants should be managed perioperatively remains an area of ongoing debate, but a disadvantage shared by all 3 is that an agent for their reversal is not yet available. Selection of an appropriate anticoagulant in patients with HF is patient-specific, and should account for both clinical and socioeconomic factors.

Combined dual antiplatelet therapy and oral anticoagulation (ie, "triple therapy") is associated with a several-fold increase in major bleeding. The combination of clopidogrel and warfarin (ie, no aspirin) in this setting has been associated

---

Table 1
Comparison of novel oral anticoagulants

Agent	Apixaban	Dabigatran	Rivaroxaban
Class	Factor Xa inhibitor	Direct thrombin inhibitor	Factor Xa inhibitor
Approved indications	(1) Stroke and systemic embolism risk reduction in nonvalvular atrial fibrillation, and (2) venous thromboembolism risk reduction after orthopedic surgery	(1) Stroke and systemic embolism risk reduction in nonvalvular atrial fibrillation, and (2) treatment of DVT/PE	(1) Stroke and systemic embolism risk reduction in nonvalvular atrial fibrillation, (2) venous thromboembolism risk reduction after orthopedic surgery, and (3) treatment of DVT/PE
Comparison with warfarin in atrial fibrillation	Superior at reducing risk of stroke and systemic embolism; lower risk of major bleeding, including intracranial bleeding	Superior at reducing risk of stroke and systemic embolism; similar risk of major bleeding, but lower risk of intracranial bleeding	Similar at reducing risk of stroke and systemic embolism; similar risk of major bleeding, but lower risk of intracranial bleeding
Elimination	27% renal	Primarily renal	Primarily renal
Half-life	12–15 h	12–17 h	5–9 h
Contraindications and precautions	Not recommended in prosthetic heart valves Combined strong CYP3A4 inhibitors and P-gp inhibitors Severe liver disease	Contraindicated in mechanical heart valves; use in other valves not recommended Advanced age (>75 y) CrCl <15 mL/min P-gp inhibitors and CrCl <30 mL/min Severe liver disease	Not recommended in prosthetic heart valves CrCl <15 mL/min Combined strong CYP3A4 inhibitors and P-gp inhibitors and inducers Moderate to severe liver disease

Abbreviations: CrCl, creatinine clearance; CYP, cytochrome P 450; DVT, deep vein thrombosis; PE, pulmonary embolism; P-gp, p-glycoprotein.

with a lower risk of bleeding, although only one-fourth of patients had HF at baseline.[36] Addition of a histamine-2 (H_2) antagonist or proton pump inhibitor (PPI) should be considered in patients at high risk for gastrointestinal bleed (eg, advanced age, concomitant use of steroids or nonsteroidal anti-inflammatory drugs, *Helicobacter pylori* infection) in whom dual antiplatelet therapy or triple therapy is indicated.[37]

Chronic Obstructive Pulmonary Disease

One of the most common therapeutic dilemmas is the underprescribing and underdosing of BB therapy in patients with chronic obstructive pulmonary disease (COPD). Bisoprolol is associated with small reductions in forced expiratory volume in 1 second (FEV_1) but no differences in response to inhaled β_2-agonist therapy, COPD symptoms, or quality of life.[38] Although carvedilol has been associated with larger reductions in FEV_1 compared with bisoprolol and metoprolol, it is usually well-tolerated in patients with COPD.[39] Thus, BB therapy should not be withheld in HF, although initiation and titration should be performed with caution, as β_1-selectivity is diminished at higher doses.

Potential drug-disease interactions have also been proposed with other HF therapies. A chronic cough is common in patients with COPD and may be mistaken for the dry cough attributed to ACEI therapy. Aggressive diuretic therapy can produce metabolic alkalosis, which may impair respiratory drive in patients with COPD.

Drugs used in the management of COPD also have been implicated in exacerbations of HF. Whether inhaled anticholinergic therapies increase cardiovascular risk remains an area of controversy, as short-acting ipratropium has been associated with risk, whereas improvements are observed with long-acting tiotropium.[40,41] Similar discrepancies exist in studies of inhaled β_2-agonists, as short-acting inhaled β_2-agonists have been associated with increases in all-cause mortality and HF hospitalization but not long-acting formulations.[42,43] Whether short-acting agents truly increase risk or simply represent more severe disease is unknown. Finally, the use of corticosteroids for COPD exacerbations may increase fluid retention in patients with HF. Although the impact is likely minimal when used for short durations (5–7 days), patients requiring longer durations may require more aggressive diuretic therapy.

Diabetes Mellitus

Clinicians have been urged to use metformin with caution in patients with HF because of a risk of lactic acidosis, despite substantial evidence to the contrary.[44] In fact, evidence suggests metformin decreases morbidity and mortality in a broad range of cardiovascular diseases, including HF.[45] Although reduced end-organ perfusion in the setting of decompensated HF may increase the risk of lactic acidosis, no prospective trials have identified metformin as a contributor. Thus, its use should not be avoided in eligible patients, and for those with decompensated HF, metformin may be temporarily withheld but should be started before discharge.

Although an increased risk of cardiovascular events with thiazolidinediones (eg, pioglitazone) remains controversial, their use in HF has been limited. Thiazolidinediones are associated with worsening edema and weight gain and have been linked to worsening HF, although studies have been inconsistent.[46] In light of their potential risks and the availability of numerous alternatives, thiazolidinediones should be avoided in HF.

Insulin also confers a poor prognosis in HF, but whether this is confounding due to disease severity or the therapy itself remains unknown.[47] In contrast, glucagonlike peptide-1 receptor agonists may confer benefits in patients with cardiovascular disease and prospective trials are ongoing.[48]

Several fundamental therapies for HF may complicate management of diabetes. Inhibitors of the renin-angiotensin-aldosterone system have been linked to higher rates of hyperkalemia in patients with diabetes. Beta blockers may impair the physiologic response to hypoglycemia and recognition of its signs and symptoms, although the clinical significance of these effects is unknown. Patients with diabetes are often less likely to receive these evidence-based therapies, but these agents should not be withheld given their well-established benefits.

Renal Dysfunction

Renal dysfunction impairs the elimination of many drugs (eg, digoxin) and presents several therapeutic dilemmas related to HF therapy. Despite the benefits of ACEI and ARBs in both HF and chronic kidney disease (CKD), underprescribing and underdosing of these agents is common and therapy is often withdrawn inappropriately during acute exacerbations of HF. An expected increase in serum creatinine of up to 30% may occur with initiation or up-titration of therapy but long-term use is associated with preservation of renal function. To improve the likelihood of successful initiation, ACEI or ARB should be initiated at lower starting doses and titrated more slowly in CKD. Additional recommendations for managing ACEI or ARB therapy have been described previously.

Loop diuretics also are often underdosed in renal dysfunction, as higher doses are required to produce adequate diuresis in both CKD and HF. Loop diuretics have been associated with worsening renal function, but it is unclear whether this is confounding due to disease severity or an actual adverse effect. In a large trial of patients with acute decompensated HF, high-dose diuretics (ie, 2.5 times outpatient dose) did not worsen the primary safety end point of renal function, although differences in some secondary safety end points were observed.[49]

As described previously, ARA therapy should be initiated cautiously in patients with renal dysfunction given an increased risk of exacerbating kidney injury and/or hyperkalemia.

Anemia and Iron Deficiency

Anemia is common in patients with HF, and although iron deficiency often contributes to anemia, it is now also recognized as a distinct clinical entity in HF. Impaired absorption and sequestration of iron may limit utility of oral iron therapies.[50,51] Substantial evidence supports the use of intravenous iron, given improvements in functional status and quality of life in both anemic and nonanemic subgroups.[51] Therefore, its use should be considered in those with evidence of iron deficiency, even in the absence of concomitant anemia. Although erythropoietin-stimulating agents (ESAs) showed early promise in the management of anemia in HF, a more recent trial demonstrated no improvement in clinical outcomes and an increase in thromboembolic events.[52] As a result, ESAs should be reserved for anemia due to conditions where their benefit is well-established (eg, CKD, cancer).

Depression

Although BBs have been implicated in worsening depression, this is not supported by evidence from clinical trials. Initiation and up-titration may cause fatigue, but these effects are often transient and not linked to worsening mood. Of the therapies used for depression, selective serotonin reuptake inhibitors (SSRIs) have the most optimal safety profile. Prolongation of the QTc interval may occur, although less commonly than with other classes of antidepressants. Although SSRIs have not been associated with improved outcomes in HF, they are the preferred first-line therapy in this population. Serotonin-norepinephrine reuptake inhibitors (eg, venlafaxine) may be considered in those with suboptimal response to SSRIs given minor and often insignificant cardiovascular adverse effects (eg, hypertension).

Tricyclic antidepressants can cause tachycardia, orthostatic hypotension, QTc prolongation, and dry mouth, which may increase thirst in patients with fluid restrictions and should not be used. Monoamine oxidase inhibitors also should be avoided. Drug-drug interactions are common, as many antidepressants are metabolized through the cytochrome P 450 (CYP450) system.

Arthritis and Gout

The management of arthritis, gout, and other rheumatologic disorders presents a number of therapeutic dilemmas in HF. Use of nonsteroidal anti-inflammatory drugs (NSAIDs) is common and is discussed in more detail later in this article. Corticosteroids should be avoided or used for only short durations given their propensity to cause fluid retention and exacerbate other comorbid conditions (eg, diabetes). Allopurinol and colchicine are generally well-tolerated, although dose adjustments may be required in patients with renal impairment. Biologic agents used in rheumatoid arthritis (eg, infliximab, a tumor necrosis factor α inhibitor) should be avoided, given their association with worsening HF. The contribution of HF therapies to the incidence of gout and other rheumatologic disorders is unclear; aggressive diuresis may worsen gout, although this may be confounded by renal dysfunction in HF.

Infectious Diseases

Exclusion of coexisting infections is challenging in HF and empiric antibiotic use is common. Antibiotics should be selected and dosed judiciously in patients with advanced HF, given its impact on drug pharmacokinetics. As a consequence, dose adjustments published in tertiary references as well as equations used to predict drug elimination may be less accurate. Certain classes of antimicrobial drugs may be especially problematic in patients with HF. The arrhythmogenic potential of macrolides and fluoroquinolones is well-established, and the volume required for drug administration (eg, vancomycin) or salt content (eg, piperacillin-tazobactam, which may provide >1 g sodium per day) may require additional diuresis in acutely decompensated patients.

The incidence of dilated cardiomyopathy due to human immunodeficiency virus (HIV) has decreased as a result of combination antiretroviral therapy (cART). However, given its success in extending survival for patients with HIV, many develop similar chronic conditions as non-HIV populations. Given the growing number of patients with HIV and HF, special attention to drug-drug interactions is necessary. Although few interactions exist with core HF therapies, common cardiovascular drugs warranting assessment include calcium channel blockers, statins, clopidogrel, digoxin, antiarrhythmics, and anticoagulants. Finally, cART therapies interact with many therapies used for comorbid conditions, and consultation with a clinical pharmacist is advised.

MEDICATIONS TO AVOID
Prescription Medications

Mechanisms for harm with prescription medications include sodium and fluid retention, neurohormonal activation, negative inotropic effects, and positive chronotropic effects. A list of prescription medications associated with harm in HF as well as recommendations for their management is provided in **Table 2**.

A therapeutic dilemma among many prescription medications is the risk of QTc prolongation and torsades de pointes. Classes of medications associated with QTc prolongation include antiarrhythmic drugs, nonsedating antihistamines, macrolide antibiotics, antifungals, antimalarials, tricyclic antidepressants, neuroleptics, and prokinetics. The risk is further compounded by coadministration of multiple QTc-prolonging medications and/or medications that inhibit their metabolism (eg, CYP3A4 inhibitors). The risk of QTc prolongation also is increased in women, patients with organic heart disease (eg, congenital long QT syndrome), electrolyte abnormalities (eg, hypokalemia, hypomagnesaemia), bradycardia, and hepatic impairment. In clinical practice, QTc-prolongation can be avoided by using recommended doses based on age and renal and/or hepatic impairment, and

---

Table 2
Prescription medications to avoid in patients with heart failure

Medication (*Mechanism of Action*)	Recommended Action
Cardiovascular agents	
Antiarrhythmic agents (Classes I and III) *Negative inotropic effects, proarrhythmic effects*	Avoid all Class I and select Class III agents (eg, ibutilide, sotalol); amiodarone or dofetilide may be considered
Aspirin *Inhibition of prostaglandins (proposed)*	Limit use primarily to those with ischemic cardiomyopathy; weigh risk of benefit vs risk in patients with nonischemic cardiomyopathy Caution in patient receiving concomitant P2Y12 inhibitors and/or warfarin; consider proton pump inhibitor therapy in patients at high risk for GI bleeding and those receiving all 3 therapies
Beta agonists *Direct positive chronotropic effect and hypokalemia promoting arrhythmias*	Avoid long-term systemic administration in patients with HF; if the inhaled route is used, long-acting agents are preferred; for both routes, use lowest effective dose
Calcium channel blockers (select) *Negative inotropic effects, neurohormonal activation*	Avoid verapamil, diltiazem, nifedipine, nisoldipine, nicardipine; use non-DHP calcium channel blockers (amlodipine, felodipine) for uncontrolled HTN and UA but only after beta-blocker dose optimized and other therapies optimized (eg, ACE inhibitor dose for HTN) or considered (eg, nitrates for UA)
Cilostazol *Inhibition of PDE III, resulting in ventricular tachycardia and PVCs*	Avoid use in patients with HF
Minoxodil *Fluid retention; stimulation of the renin-angiotensin-aldosterone system*	Avoid use in patients with HF
Pentoxifylline *Methylxanthine derivative, which may produce dyspnea, edema, hypotension, angina, and palpitations/arrhythmia*	Avoid in patients with HF

(continued on next page)

Table 2
(continued)

Medication (*Mechanism of Action*)	Recommended Action
Chemotherapeutic agents	
Anthracyline agents (eg, doxorubicin, daunorubicin, mitoxantrone)[a] *Cumulative dose-dependent cardiotoxicity; multiple proposed mechanisms for direct cardiotoxic effects*	May present as early or late onset; noninvasive cardiac monitoring recommended; use of anthracycline analogues of comparable efficacy and less cardiotoxicity whenever possible; use cardioprotective therapy (dexrazoxane) when indicated
HER2/Neu agents (eg, trastuzumab, pertuzumab) *Loss of erbB2-mediated signaling which interferes with the heart's ability to respond to stress*	Close cardiac monitoring must be performed for all patients receiving anti-HER2 agents; primarily asymptomatic LV dysfunction; likely reversible with discontinuation and restoration of erbB2-mediated signaling
Neuropsychiatric agents	
Amphetamines *Peripheral sympathetic agonist activity, tachycardia, arrhythmias*	Avoid use in patients with HF
Carbamazepine *Negative inotropic and chronotropic effects; suppression of SNA and AVC; anticholinergic effects accelerating the formation of reentry circuits*	Avoid use in patients with HF if possible; use other first line therapies for seizures, depression, and affective disorders
Clozapine *Mechanism unknown*	Actively monitor for new or increased HF symptoms
Tricyclic antidepressants *Negative inotropic effects; increase in automaticity; slowing of intracardiac conduction; proarrhythmic properties*	Avoid if possible in patients with HF; use other first-line agents for depression and neuropathy
Other	
Glucocorticoids *Sodium/fluid retention*	Active monitoring for new or increased HF symptoms; conservative use with the lowest doses needed for efficacy
Itraconazole *Negative inotropic activity*	Avoid administration for onychomycosis; use caution and increase monitoring for signs or symptoms of HF in the treatment of systemic fungal infections
Nonsteroidal anti-inflammatory agents *Sodium and water retention; blunted response to exogenous diuretics; increased systemic vascular resistance*	Avoid use in patients with symptomatic LV dysfunction if possible Use ASA 81 mg/d only as needed for ASCVD or CVD
Thiazolidinediones *Fluid retention*	Avoid use in patients with HF or at high risk for developing HF

Abbreviations: ACE, angiotensin-converting enzyme; ASA, aspirin; ASCVD, atherosclerotic cardiovascular disease; AVC, atrioventricular conduction; CVD, cerebrovascular disease; DHP, dihydropyridine; GI, gastrointestinal; HF, heart failure; HTN, hypertension; LV, left ventricular; PDE, phosphodiesterase; PVC, premature ventricular complexes; SNA, sinus nodal automaticity; UA, unstable angina.

[a] Other less commonly cited cardiotoxic chemotherapeutic agents: cyclophosphamide, ifosfamide, mitomycin and fluorouracil.

Data from Amabile CM, Spencer AP. Keeping your patient with heart failure safe: a review of potentially dangerous medications. Arch Intern Med 2004;164(7):709–20. http://dx.doi.org/10.1001/archinte.164.7.709.

avoiding use of QTc-prolonging medications in at-risk patients. Coadministration of medications that can prolong the QTc interval, CYP450 inhibitors (eg, imidazole antifungals, macrolide antibiotics), and therapies known to cause electrolyte disturbances should be avoided. Serum potassium and magnesium concentrations should be evaluated regularly, especially in patients receiving diuretics. Furthermore, electrocardiograms should be routinely performed before and after initiation or titration of a QTc-prolonging medication.

Nonprescription Medications

Use of nonprescription medications in patients with HF may be as high as 93%, and patients taking them are more likely to be older, Caucasian, and be under the care of a cardiologist.[53] Importantly, only 5% of patients report using nonprescription medications to replace one or more of their prescription medications, although it is often not clear to patients what constitutes a nonprescription medication. Use of full-strength aspirin, iron, antihistamines, decongestants, antidiarrheal agents, sodium-based antacids and salt substitutes is frequent (**Table 3**), and the potential harm associated with these medications in HF is described in **Table 4**. Similarly concerning is that only approximately 50% of patients report consulting a pharmacist before using nonprescription therapies.[54]

Although some NSAIDs are available by prescription, most are readily available to the consumer as nonprescription medications. Although cyclooxygenase-2 (COX-2) inhibitors and traditional NSAIDs are equally efficacious in their analgesic and anti-inflammatory properties, the risk of

gastrointestinal ulcers and bleeding is less with COX-2 inhibitors. However, these agents may also carry an increased risk of major adverse cardiovascular events. In fact, 2 COX-2 inhibitors, rofecoxib (Vioxx) and valdecoxib (Bextra), were removed from the market because of concerns of increased risk of heart attacks or stroke. Although a large meta-analysis found up to a 5 mm Hg increase in mean blood pressure with NSAIDs, only a minimal change has been observed with ibuprofen or naproxen.[55,56]

Overall, NSAIDs are known to adversely affect patients with HF, and should be avoided or withdrawn whenever possible.[1] Their use has been associated with an increased risk of death and hospitalization due to HF or myocardial infarction; these effects appear to be mediated by both NSAID dose and half-life but not COX-selectivity.[57–59] Although ibuprofen and naproxen are thought to be less cardiotoxic, an increased risk of mortality and hospitalization has been observed with higher doses (ibuprofen >1200 mg/d, naproxen >500 mg/d).[60]

Use of nonprescription medications with stimulant properties should also be avoided if possible. These include decongestants (available in many combination cold products), weight-loss supplements, or agents containing caffeine (eg, No-Doz). Although adverse effects have been observed with pseudoephedrine, further studies are needed to confirm if phenylephrine carries the same risk. Safer alternatives for patients with congestion include nasal decongestants, which have less systemic absorption, or saline nasal spray. Although nonprescription anorectics are safer following the removal of ephedra, many contain caffeine. A statistically significant J-shaped relationship between coffee consumption and HF has been observed, with a decreased risk at 4 cups per day and increased risks at higher levels of consumption.[61]

Both laxatives and antacids are associated with hypermagnesemia, which may be increased in patients with HF due to comorbid renal dysfunction or impaired motility. One study of elderly patients with HF demonstrated a significant association between hypermagnesemia and antacid or laxative use, and reduced survival among those who were hypermagnesemic.[62] Additionally, the sodium content of antacids may approach 0.3 to 0.9 g per dose, with directions allowing for administration of up to 4 to 8 doses per day. Nonprescription H_2 antagonists and PPIs are implicated in numerous drug interactions, and PPIs carry an added risk of bone loss due to altered calcium absorption.

Potassium-containing salt substitutes have perhaps the greatest potential to cause harm in

Table 3
Frequency of nonprescription medication use in patients with heart failure patients

Nonprescription Medications	Frequency of Use, %
Low-dose aspirin, full-strength aspirin	48, 14
Acetaminophen	47
Vitamins	46
Antacid: nonsodium based	26
Laxatives	16
Nonsteroidal anti-inflammatory drugs	13
Iron	12
Antihistamine/Decongestant	7–8
Antidiarrheal	8
Sleeping aid	5
Salt substitute	4

Agents used less than 2%: sodium-based antacids, cough suppressants, motion sickness aids, smoking cessation aids, weight control aids, other.

Data from Albert NM, Rathman L, Ross D, et al. Predictors of over-the-counter drug and herbal therapies use in elderly patients with heart failure. J Card Fail 2009;15(7):600–6.

Table 4
Nonprescription medications to avoid in patients with heart failure

Nonprescription Medication	Potential Harm in Heart Failure
Laxatives	Risk of dehydration and related electrolyte disturbances Drug-drug interactions (bulk-forming laxatives) Hypermagnesemia (hyperosmotic saline laxatives)
Antacids	Drug-drug interactions Sodium content Hypermagnesemia
Antihistamines	Impaired motility Tachycardia, palpitations
Decongestants (eg, pseudoephedrine, phenylephrine[a])	Increased systemic vascular resistance Increased blood pressure Tachycardia, arrhythmia
Antidiarrheals	Drug interactions Bismuth subsalicylate (eg, Pepto-Bismol, Kaopectate)
Weight-control aids	Limited concern since ban of ephedra-containing products; however, many aids contain caffeine (see next item)
Caffeine (eg, No-Doz, energy drinks/shots)	Risk with high levels of consumption (>4 servings/day)

[a] Documented reports of myocardial infarction, stroke, arrhythmia with pseudoephedrine. Additional studies needed with phenylephrine.

patients with HF because of an increased risk of hyperkalemia with ACEI, ARB, and/or ARA therapy. Patients should be counseled to limit the use of these products to avoid an increased risk of arrhythmias.

Complementary and Alternative Medicine

Nonprescription medications also include vitamins, minerals, and complementary and alternative medicines (CAM). Among patients with HF, the use of vitamins or minerals (48%) and herbals (38%) is second only to pain relievers (59%).[63] Of patients who reported they would avoid herbal supplements (71%), 21% were routinely taking one. Although most nonprescription medications are under regulatory oversight, evidence of safety and/or efficacy is not required for vitamins, minerals, or CAM.

Malnutrition and micronutrient deficiency is common in patients with HF because of reduced intake, increased wasting, and diuretic therapy. Low concentrations of thiamine, selenium, and zinc, as well as elevated copper, have been associated with reduced LVEF or other measures of HF severity. Factors contributing to nutritional deficiencies in HF include reduced hunger, dietary restrictions, fatigue, nausea, anxiety, sadness, reduced absorption, increased urinary loss, and increased consumption due to oxidative stress. To date, few interventional studies have been conducted and are limited in sample size.[64,65] The largest and most robust trials to date have involved vitamin E, and demonstrated either no benefit or increased risk for the development of HF.[66–68] Caution should be exerted with large quantities of vitamin supplementation.

Potential adverse effects of common CAM therapies include sympathomimetic effects (eg, ma huang, yohimbe), excess aldosterone or glucocorticoid release (eg, licorice), platelet dysfunction (eg, dan shen, garlic, ginkgo), and coumarinlike effects (eg, aescin, dong quai).[69] Drug-drug interactions may also occur, with St John's Wort being well documented in the literature. Because CAM therapies do not undergo regulatory oversight, they are rarely evaluated for their potential to cause drug-drug interactions.

Drug-Drug Interactions

The primary mechanism by which drug-drug interactions occur in patients with HF is altered pharmacokinetics. Altered gastric pH will increase absorption of weak acids and reduce absorption for weak bases. Interactions involving metabolic function may alter serum drug concentrations depending on whether metabolism is enhanced or inhibited; these effects may be even further complicated if active metabolites are involved. Other mechanisms also exist (**Table 5**). Most notable are pharmacodynamic drug interactions, which involve additive effects (eg, bradycardia

Table 5
Common drug interactions observed in patients with heart failure

Drug/Class	Mechanism	Example
Amiodarone	Reduced metabolism	↑ Digoxin, ↑ simvastatin, ↑ warfarin
Antacids	Increased gastric pH Chelation	↑ Digoxin, glyburide ↓ Antibiotics (select)
Digoxin	Reduced absorption Reduced metabolism/excretion	Kaolin-pectin, cholestyramine, antacids (↓ digoxin) Amiodarone, oral antibiotics, propafenone, quinidine, ranolazine (↑ digoxin)
H2-antagonists[a]	Reduced metabolism	↓ Warfarin, select beta-blockers (eg, metoprolol), DHP calcium blockers, lidocaine, quinidine
Hydrochlorothiazide	Reduced renal tubular secretion	↑ Dofetilide
Proton pump inhibitors	Reduced activation Reduced metabolism	↓ Clopidogrel[b] ↑ Tacrolimus, cyclosporine, fluvoxamine
Phosphodiesterase inhibitors	Excessive nitric oxide release	Nitrates – excessive hypotension
Ranolazine	Reduced metabolism	↑ Digoxin, limit simvastatin dose to 20 mg/d, limit dose of lovastatin and metformin in select patients; contraindicated with strong CYP3A4 inhibitors and inducers, including St John's Wort

Abbreviations: ↑, increase; ↓, decrease; CYP, cytochrome P 450; DHP, dihydropyridine.
[a] Specific for cimetidine (Tagamet).
[b] Theoretical with omeprazole (Prilosec) and lansoprazole (Prevacid).

with BB and digoxin, hyperkalemia with ACEI and ARA). Although many of these interactions require only dose or frequency adjustment (ie, spacing antacid administration around an interacting therapy), select interactions require complete avoidance to minimize lack of efficacy or increased risk of toxicity.

REFERENCES

1. Yancy CW, Jessup M, Bozkurt B, et al. 2013 ACCF/AHA guideline for the management of heart failure: a report of the American College of Cardiology Foundation/American Heart Association Task Force on Practice Guidelines. J Am Coll Cardiol 2013; 62(16):e147–239. http://dx.doi.org/10.1016/j.jacc.2013.05.019.

2. Pitt B, Poole-Wilson PA, Segal R, et al. Effect of losartan compared with captopril on mortality in patients with symptomatic heart failure: randomised trial—the Losartan Heart Failure Survival Study ELITE II. Lancet 2000;355(9215):1582–7.

3. Granger CB, McMurray JJ, Yusuf S, et al. Effects of candesartan in patients with chronic heart failure and reduced left-ventricular systolic function intolerant to angiotensin-converting-enzyme inhibitors: the CHARM-Alternative trial. Lancet 2003; 362(9386):772–6. http://dx.doi.org/10.1016/S0140-6736(03)14284-5.

4. Packer M, Poole-Wilson PA, Armstrong PW, et al. Comparative effects of low and high doses of the angiotensin-converting enzyme inhibitor, lisinopril, on morbidity and mortality in chronic heart failure. ATLAS Study Group. Circulation 1999;100(23): 2312–8.

5. Konstam MA, Neaton JD, Dickstein K, et al. Effects of high-dose versus low-dose losartan on clinical outcomes in patients with heart failure (HEAAL study): a randomised, double-blind trial. Lancet 2009;374(9704):1840–8. http://dx.doi.org/10.1016/S0140-6736(09)61913-9.

6. Bristow MR, Gilbert EM, Abraham WT, et al. Carvedilol produces dose-related improvements in left ventricular function and survival in subjects with chronic heart failure. MOCHA Investigators. Circulation 1996;94(11):2807–16.

7. Packer M, Bristow MR, Cohn JN, et al. The effect of carvedilol on morbidity and mortality in patients with chronic heart failure. U.S. Carvedilol Heart Failure Study Group. N Engl J Med

1996;334(21):1349–55. http://dx.doi.org/10.1056/NEJM199605233342101.

8. Effect of metoprolol CR/XL in chronic heart failure: Metoprolol CR/XL Randomised Intervention Trial in Congestive Heart Failure (MERIT-HF). Lancet 1999;353(9169):2001–7.

9. The Cardiac Insufficiency Bisoprolol Study II (CIBIS-II): a randomised trial. Lancet 1999;353(9146):9–13.

10. Kubo T, Azevedo ER, Newton GE, et al. Lack of evidence for peripheral alpha(1)- adrenoceptor blockade during long-term treatment of heart failure with carvedilol. J Am Coll Cardiol 2001;38(5):1463–9.

11. Wikstrand J, Hjalmarson A, Waagstein F, et al. Dose of metoprolol CR/XL and clinical outcomes in patients with heart failure: analysis of the experience in metoprolol CR/XL randomized intervention trial in chronic heart failure (MERIT-HF). J Am Coll Cardiol 2002;40(3):491–8.

12. Simon T, Mary-Krause M, Funck-Brentano C, et al. Bisoprolol dose-response relationship in patients with congestive heart failure: a subgroup analysis in the cardiac insufficiency bisoprolol study(CIBIS II). Eur Heart J 2003;24(6):552–9.

13. Pitt B, Zannad F, Remme WJ, et al. The effect of spironolactone on morbidity and mortality in patients with severe heart failure. Randomized Aldactone Evaluation Study Investigators. N Engl J Med 1999;341(10):709–17. http://dx.doi.org/10.1056/NEJM199909023411001.

14. Zannad F, McMurray JJ, Krum H, et al. Eplerenone in patients with systolic heart failure and mild symptoms. N Engl J Med 2011;364(1):11–21. http://dx.doi.org/10.1056/NEJMoa1009492.

15. Phelan D, Thavendiranathan P, Collier P, et al. Aldosterone antagonists improve ejection fraction and functional capacity independently of functional class: a meta-analysis of randomised controlled trials. Heart 2012;98(23):1693–700. http://dx.doi.org/10.1136/heartjnl-2012-302178.

16. Taylor AL, Ziesche S, Yancy C, et al. Combination of isosorbide dinitrate and hydralazine in blacks with heart failure. N Engl J Med 2004;351(20):2049–57. http://dx.doi.org/10.1056/NEJMoa042934.

17. Anand IS, Tam SW, Rector TS, et al. Influence of blood pressure on the effectiveness of a fixed-dose combination of isosorbide dinitrate and hydralazine in the African-American Heart Failure Trial. J Am Coll Cardiol 2007;49(1):32–9. http://dx.doi.org/10.1016/j.jacc.2006.04.109.

18. Digitalis Investigation Group. The effect of digoxin on mortality and morbidity in patients with heart failure. N Engl J Med 1997;336(8):525–33. http://dx.doi.org/10.1056/NEJM199702203360801.

19. Adams KF Jr, Patterson JH, Gattis WA, et al. Relationship of serum digoxin concentration to mortality and morbidity in women in the digitalis investigation group trial: a retrospective analysis. J Am Coll Cardiol 2005;46(3):497–504. http://dx.doi.org/10.1016/j.jacc.2005.02.091.

20. Gissi-HF Investigators, Tavazzi L, Maggioni AP, et al. Effect of n-3 polyunsaturated fatty acids in patients with chronic heart failure (the GISSI-HF trial): a randomised, double-blind, placebo-controlled trial. Lancet 2008;372(9645):1223–30. http://dx.doi.org/10.1016/S0140-6736(08)61239-8.

21. Nodari S, Triggiani M, Campia U, et al. Effects of n-3 polyunsaturated fatty acids on left ventricular function and functional capacity in patients with dilated cardiomyopathy. J Am Coll Cardiol 2011;57(7):870–9. http://dx.doi.org/10.1016/j.jacc.2010.11.017.

22. McMurray JJ, Ostergren J, Swedberg K, et al. Effects of candesartan in patients with chronic heart failure and reduced left-ventricular systolic function taking angiotensin-converting-enzyme inhibitors: the CHARM-Added trial. Lancet 2003;362(9386):767–71. http://dx.doi.org/10.1016/S0140-6736(03)14283-3.

23. Makani H, Bangalore S, Desouza KA, et al. Efficacy and safety of dual blockade of the renin-angiotensin system: meta-analysis of randomised trials. BMJ 2013;346:f360.

24. Gheorghiade M, Böhm M, Greene SJ, et al. Effect of aliskiren on postdischarge mortality and heart failure readmissions among patients hospitalized for heart failure: the ASTRONAUT randomized trial. JAMA 2013;309(11):1125–35. http://dx.doi.org/10.1001/jama.2013.1954.

25. Wong CY, Chaudhry SI, Desai MM, et al. Trends in comorbidity, disability, and polypharmacy in heart failure. Am J Med 2011;124(2):136–43. http://dx.doi.org/10.1016/j.amjmed.2010.08.017.

26. Braunstein JB, Anderson GF, Gerstenblith G, et al. Noncardiac comorbidity increases preventable hospitalizations and mortality among Medicare beneficiaries with chronic heart failure. J Am Coll Cardiol 2003;42(7):1226–33.

27. Cleland JG, Findlay I, Jafri S, et al. The Warfarin/Aspirin Study in Heart failure (WASH): a randomized trial comparing antithrombotic strategies for patients with heart failure. Am Heart J 2004;148(1):157–64. http://dx.doi.org/10.1016/j.ahj.2004.03.010.

28. Massie BM, Collins JF, Ammon SE, et al. Randomized trial of warfarin, aspirin, and clopidogrel in patients with chronic heart failure: the Warfarin and Antiplatelet Therapy in Chronic Heart Failure (WATCH) trial. Circulation 2009;119(12):1616–24. http://dx.doi.org/10.1161/CIRCULATIONAHA.108.801753.

29. Homma S, Thompson JL, Pullicino PM, et al. Warfarin and aspirin in patients with heart failure and sinus rhythm. N Engl J Med 2012;366(20):1859–69. http://dx.doi.org/10.1056/NEJMoa1202299.

30. Antithrombotic Trialists' (ATT) Collaboration, Baigent C, Blackwell L, et al. Aspirin in the primary and secondary prevention of vascular disease: collaborative meta-analysis of individual participant data from randomised trials. Lancet 2009;373(9678): 1849–60. http://dx.doi.org/10.1016/S0140-6736(09) 60503-1.

31. Wiviott SD, Braunwald E, McCabe CH, et al. Prasugrel versus clopidogrel in patients with acute coronary syndromes. N Engl J Med 2007;357(20):2001–15. http://dx.doi.org/10.1056/NEJMoa0706482.

32. Wallentin L, Becker RC, Budaj A, et al. Ticagrelor versus clopidogrel in patients with acute coronary syndromes. N Engl J Med 2009;361(11):1045–57. http://dx.doi.org/10.1056/NEJMoa0904327.

33. Granger CB, Alexander JH, McMurray JJ, et al. Apixaban versus warfarin in patients with atrial fibrillation. N Engl J Med 2011;365(11):981–92. http://dx.doi.org/10.1056/NEJMoa1107039.

34. Connolly SJ, Ezekowitz MD, Yusuf S, et al. Dabigatran versus warfarin in patients with atrial fibrillation. N Engl J Med 2009;361(12):1139–51. http://dx.doi.org/10.1056/NEJMoa0905561.

35. Patel MR, Mahaffey KW, Garg J, et al. Rivaroxaban versus warfarin in nonvalvular atrial fibrillation. N Engl J Med 2011;365(10):883–91. http://dx.doi.org/10.1056/NEJMoa1009638.

36. Dewilde WJ, Oirbans T, Verheugt FW, et al. Use of clopidogrel with or without aspirin in patients taking oral anticoagulant therapy and undergoing percutaneous coronary intervention: an open-label, randomised, controlled trial. Lancet 2013;381(9872): 1107–15. http://dx.doi.org/10.1016/S0140-6736(12) 62177-1.

37. Bhatt DL, Scheiman J, Abraham NS, et al. ACCF/ACG/AHA 2008 expert consensus document on reducing the gastrointestinal risks of antiplatelet therapy and NSAID use: a report of the American College of Cardiology Foundation Task Force on Clinical Expert Consensus Documents. Circulation 2008;118(18):1894–909. http://dx.doi.org/10.1161/CIRCULATIONAHA.108.191087.

38. Hawkins NM, MacDonald MR, Petrie MC, et al. Bisoprolol in patients with heart failure and moderate to severe chronic obstructive pulmonary disease: a randomized controlled trial. Eur J Heart Fail 2009;11(7): 684–90. http://dx.doi.org/10.1093/eurjhf/hfp066.

39. Jabbour A, Macdonald PS, Keogh AM, et al. Differences between beta-blockers in patients with chronic heart failure and chronic obstructive pulmonary disease: a randomized crossover trial. J Am Coll Cardiol 2010;55(17):1780–7. http://dx.doi.org/10.1016/j.jacc.2010.01.024.

40. Ogale SS, Lee TA, Au DH, et al. Cardiovascular events associated with ipratropium bromide in COPD. Chest 2010;137(1):13–9. http://dx.doi.org/10.1378/chest.08-2367.

41. Celli B, Decramer M, Leimer I, et al. Cardiovascular safety of tiotropium in patients with COPD. Chest 2010;137(1):20–30. http://dx.doi.org/10.1378/chest.09-0011.

42. Au DH, Udris EM, Fan VS, et al. Risk of mortality and heart failure exacerbations associated with inhaled beta-adrenoceptor agonists among patients with known left ventricular systolic dysfunction. Chest 2003;123(6):1964–9.

43. Calverley PM, Anderson JA, Celli B, et al. Salmeterol and fluticasone propionate and survival in chronic obstructive pulmonary disease. N Engl J Med 2007;356(8):775–89. http://dx.doi.org/10.1056/NEJMoa063070.

44. Salpeter SR, Greyber E, Pasternak GA, et al. Risk of fatal and nonfatal lactic acidosis with metformin use in type 2 diabetes mellitus. Cochrane Database Syst Rev 2010;(4):CD002967. http://dx.doi.org/10.1002/14651858.CD002967.pub4.

45. Eurich DT, Majumdar SR, McAlister FA, et al. Improved clinical outcomes associated with metformin in patients with diabetes and heart failure. Diabetes Care 2005;28(10):2345–51.

46. Karter AJ, Ahmed AT, Liu J, et al. Pioglitazone initiation and subsequent hospitalization for congestive heart failure. Diabet Med 2005;22(8):986–93. http://dx.doi.org/10.1111/j.1464-5491.2005.01704.x.

47. Smooke S, Horwich TB, Fonarow GC. Insulin-treated diabetes is associated with a marked increase in mortality in patients with advanced heart failure. Am Heart J 2005;149(1):168–74. http://dx.doi.org/10.1016/j.ahj.2004.07.005.

48. Burgmaier M, Heinrich C, Marx N. Cardiovascular effects of GLP-1 and GLP-1-based therapies: implications for the cardiovascular continuum in diabetes? Diabet Med 2013;30(3):289–99. http://dx.doi.org/10.1111/j.1464-5491.2012.03746.x.

49. Felker GM, Lee KL, Bull DA, et al. Diuretic strategies in patients with acute decompensated heart failure. N Engl J Med 2011;364(9):797–805. http://dx.doi.org/10.1056/NEJMoa1005419.

50. Beck-da-Silva L, Piardi D, Soder S, et al. IRON-HF study: a randomized trial to assess the effects of iron in heart failure patients with anemia. Int J Cardiol 2013;168(4):3439–42. http://dx.doi.org/10.1016/j.ijcard.2013.04.181.

51. Anker SD, Comin Colet J, Filippatos G, et al. Ferric carboxymaltose in patients with heart failure and iron deficiency. N Engl J Med 2009;361(25):2436–48. http://dx.doi.org/10.1056/NEJMoa0908355.

52. Swedberg K, Young JB, Anand IS, et al. Treatment of anemia with darbepoetin alfa in systolic heart failure. N Engl J Med 2013;368(13):1210–9. http://dx.doi.org/10.1056/NEJMoa1214865.

53. Albert NM, Rathman L, Ross D, et al. Predictors of over-the-counter drug and herbal therapies use in elderly patients with heart failure.

J Card Fail 2009;15(7):600–6. http://dx.doi.org/10.1016/j.cardfail.2009.02.001.

54. Pharand C, Ackman ML, Jackevicius CA, et al, Canadian Cardiovascular Pharmacists Network. Use of OTC and herbal products in patients with cardiovascular disease. Ann Pharmacother 2003;37(6):899–904.

55. Johnson AG, Nguyen TV, Day RO. Do nonsteroidal anti-inflammatory drugs affect blood pressure? A meta-analysis. Ann Intern Med 1994;121(4):289–300.

56. Sowers JR, White WB, Pitt B, et al. The effects of cyclooxygenase-2 inhibitors and nonsteroidal anti-inflammatory therapy on 24-hour blood pressure in patients with hypertension, osteoarthritis, and type 2 diabetes mellitus. Arch Intern Med 2005;165(2):161–8. http://dx.doi.org/10.1001/archinte.165.2.161.

57. Page J, Henry D. Consumption of NSAIDs and the development of congestive heart failure in elderly patients: an underrecognized public health problem. Arch Intern Med 2000;160(6):777–84.

58. Heerdink ER, Leufkens HG, Herings RM, et al. NSAIDs associated with increased risk of congestive heart failure in elderly patients taking diuretics. Arch Intern Med 1998;158(10):1108–12.

59. Mamdani M, Juurlink DN, Lee DS, et al. Cyclo-oxygenase-2 inhibitors versus non-selective non-steroidal anti-inflammatory drugs and congestive heart failure outcomes in elderly patients: a population-based cohort study. Lancet 2004;363(9423):1751–6. http://dx.doi.org/10.1016/S0140-6736(04)16299-5.

60. Gislason GH, Rasmussen JN, Abildstrom SZ, et al. Increased mortality and cardiovascular morbidity associated with use of nonsteroidal anti-inflammatory drugs in chronic heart failure. Arch Intern Med 2009;169(2):141–9. http://dx.doi.org/10.1001/archinternmed.2008.525.

61. Mostofsky E, Rice MS, Levitan EB, et al. Habitual coffee consumption and risk of heart failure: a dose-response meta-analysis. Circ Heart Fail 2012;5(4):401–5. http://dx.doi.org/10.1161/CIRCHEARTFAILURE.112.967299.

62. Corbi G, Acanfora D, Iannuzzi GL, et al. Hypermagnesemia predicts mortality in elderly with congestive heart disease: relationship with laxative and antacid use. Rejuvenation Res 2008;11(1):129–38. http://dx.doi.org/10.1089/rej.2007.0583.

63. Ackman ML, Campbell JB, Buzak KA, et al. Use of nonprescription medications by patients with congestive heart failure. Ann Pharmacother 1999;33(6):674–9.

64. Krim SR, Campbell P, Lavie CJ, et al. Micronutrients in chronic heart failure. Curr Heart Fail Rep 2013;10(1):46–53. http://dx.doi.org/10.1007/s11897-012-0118-4.

65. McKeag NA, McKinley MC, Woodside JV, et al. The role of micronutrients in heart failure. J Acad Nutr Diet 2012;112(6):870–86. http://dx.doi.org/10.1016/j.jand.2012.01.016.

66. Yusuf S, Dagenais G, Pogue J, et al. Vitamin E supplementation and cardiovascular events in high-risk patients. The Heart Outcomes Prevention Evaluation Study Investigators. N Engl J Med 2000;342(3):154–60. http://dx.doi.org/10.1056/NEJM200001203420302.

67. Lonn E, Bosch J, Yusuf S, et al. Effects of long-term vitamin E supplementation on cardiovascular events and cancer: a randomized controlled trial. JAMA 2005;293(11):1338–47. http://dx.doi.org/10.1001/jama.293.11.1338.

68. Marchioli R, Levantesi G, Macchia A, et al. Vitamin E increases the risk of developing heart failure after myocardial infarction: results from the GISSI-Prevenzione trial. J Cardiovasc Med (Hagerstown) 2006;7(5):347–50. http://dx.doi.org/10.2459/01.JCM.0000223257.09062.17.

69. Amabile CM, Spencer AP. Keeping your patient with heart failure safe: a review of potentially dangerous medications. Arch Intern Med 2004;164(7):709–20. http://dx.doi.org/10.1001/archinte.164.7.709.

Management Strategies for Heart Failure with Preserved Ejection Fraction

Ali Vazir, MB BS, PhD, MRCP[a,b], Scott D. Solomon, MD[a],*

KEYWORDS

- Heart failure • Preserved ejection fraction • LCZ696

KEY POINTS

- The management of HFpEF is challenging and requires an accurate diagnosis. Although currently there is no convincing therapy that can prolong survival in patients with HFpEF, treatment of fluid retention and of comorbidities, such as hypertension, myocardial ischemia, and atrial fibrillation, may improve symptoms and quality of life.
- Spironolactone may be considered in patients with HFpEF with an elevated BNP, and if prescribed, patients require monitoring of potassium levels and renal function.
- Future outcome trials of HFpEF testing the efficacy of promising new agents, such as LCZ696, will have better characterization of patient phenotype to maximize the potential response to therapies.

INTRODUCTION

Epidemiologic studies have shown that approximately half of patients with heart failure (HF) have normal or near normal ejection fraction (EF); this syndrome is referred to as HF with preserved EF (HFpEF).[1–3] The overall cost of HF was estimated to be more than $30 billion for 2012,[4] and the prevalence and cost are predicted to rise with the aging population. The epidemiologic and etiologic profile of HFpEF seems to differ from that of HF with reduced EF (HFrEF), such that HFpEF patients are frequently older, more often women, obese, suffer from hypertension and atrial fibrillation, and less likely to suffer from coronary artery disease.[1–3] The risk of mortality and readmission is similar to that of HFrEF, although in trials mortality rate seems to be lower.[5] In contrast to HFrEF, there are no therapies that have been proved to improve mortality and morbidity in patients with HFpEF as acknowledged in international guidelines.[6,7] The latter relate to uncertainties surrounding the pathophysiology of HFpEF and lack of consensus of its definition and classification, which at present seems to comprise patients with heterogeneous phenotype. The specific criteria for HFpEF continue to be debated. Although all agree that EF needs to be in the "preserved" range, the cutoff ranges from 40% to 50% in various guidelines and reviews. In addition to EF in the preserved range, most guidelines require evidence of structural or functional abnormality of the heart (eg, enlarged left atrium; left ventricular [LV] hypertrophy; and/or diastolic dysfunction, such as raised E/e' ratio) in the presence of typical symptoms (eg, breathlessness) and signs (eg, raised jugular venous pressure, edema) of HF. Because these symptoms are nonspecific it is also important to exclude other potential diagnoses that may have a similar presentation.[6,7] Interestingly, in most recent trials of HFpEF, the cutoff value of EF used is 45%.

[a] Cardiovascular Division, Brigham and Women's Hospital, Harvard Medical School, 75 Francis Street, Boston, MA 02115, USA; [b] Royal Brompton Hospital, Royal Brompton and Harefield NHS Foundation Trust, NIHR Cardiovascular Biomedical Research Unit and Institute of Cardiovascular Medicine and Sciences (ICMS), National Heart and Lung Institute (NHLI), Imperial College London, London, UK
* Corresponding author.
E-mail address: ssolomon@rics.bwh.harvard.edu

Heart Failure Clin 10 (2014) 591–598
http://dx.doi.org/10.1016/j.hfc.2014.07.004
1551-7136/14/$ – see front matter © 2014 Elsevier Inc. All rights reserved.

This article provides the reader with the current management strategies available for HFpEF, gives an overview of previous trials that have failed to prove the benefit of therapies to improve outcomes, and highlights promising novel therapies.

MANAGEMENT GOALS

There is no convincing therapy available to prolong survival in patients with HFpEF. Therefore, the goal of therapy is to relieve symptoms and improve quality of life. As recommended by international guidelines[6,7] this is best accomplished by treating fluid retention; reducing high ventricular rates; maintaining and restoring atrial contraction; and optimizing treatment of comorbidities, such as systemic hypertension, myocardial ischemia, diabetes mellitus, chronic obstructive lung disease, and sleep apnea (**Table 1**).

Treatment of Fluid Retention

Diuretic agents are used to treat pulmonary congestion and peripheral edema, as they are in HFrEF. The main agents used include loop diuretics and thiazide or thiazide-like drugs. The evidence base for the use of diuretics, however, is limited. The DOSE, which was the largest prospective, double-blind, randomized acute decompensated HF trial to evaluate initial diuretic strategies in patients with acute decompensated HF included a small proportion of patients with HFpEF; however, the mean LVEF was approximately 35 ± 18%. In this trial there no significant differences in either of the coprimary end points of global assessment of symptoms or change in serum creatinine over 72 hours with diuretic administration by bolus or continuous infusion or with a low- versus a high-dose strategy.

A recent study has also shown that ultrafiltration is well tolerated in patients with HFpEF and evidence of fluid retention when compared with those with HFrEF.[8] The exact role of ultrafiltration in the management of decompensated HF remains unclear, but could be considered as outlined in international guidelines.[6,7]

In general, careful attention for symptoms and signs (eg, dizziness, syncope, hypotension) of low cardiac output is necessary, because excessive preload reduction with diuretics (or nitrates or calcium antagonist) can lead to underfilling of the LV and also dynamic LV outflow tract obstruction leading to low stroke volume and low cardiac output state and hypotension. This is especially seen in patients with excessive LV hypertrophy with small ventricles and those with hypertrophic cardiomyopathy.

Maintenance and Restoration of Atrial Contraction

Patients with HFpEF do not tolerate atrial fibrillation, especially when the ventricular rate is high, because loss of atrial contraction can significantly reduce LV filling and therefore cardiac output. Ideally sinus rhythm should be restored and if not possible the focus should be on ventricular rate control with β-blockers, rate-lowering calcium antagonists, or digoxin.[6] Sinus rhythm may be restored with medications or electrical cardioversion. Radiofrequency ablation may also be considered. Importantly, patients with paroxysmal, persistent, or permanent atrial fibrillation should be anticoagulated if not contraindicated[6,7] to avoid risk of systemic embolization.

Optimization and Treatment of Comorbidities

The treatment of comorbidities needs to be optimized because the burden of poorly controlled comorbidity increases risk of readmission.[9] Treatment of elevated systolic and diastolic blood pressure is important, because lowering blood pressure is associated with reduced risk of developing HF in patients with hypertension.[10,11] The agents that may be used include angiotensin receptor blockers (ARB), angiotensin-converting enzyme

Table 1
Management goals for heart failure with preserved ejection fraction

Goal	Treatment Options
Treat fluid retention	Diuretics Ultrafiltration
Maintain and restore atrial contraction and rate control	Medically cardiovert with class I, II, or III antiarrhythmics β-Blocker, digoxin, rate-limiting calcium antagonists DC cardioversion Radiofrequency ablation
Optimize and treat comorbidities	Hypertension Myocardial ischemia Obstructive sleep apnea Obesity Diabetes mellitus Renal dysfunction Chronic obstructive pulmonary disease Iron deficiency
Entrance into chronic heart failure management program	Patient education Follow-up by health care team

(ACE) inhibitors, calcium antagonists, thiazide diuretics, and β-blockers. These agents have been associated with regression of LV hypertrophy, which in itself is associated with the development of diastolic dysfunction.[12] Therefore, regression of LV hypertrophy is considered to be an important treatment target; however, in the hypertension population regression of LV hypertrophy has not been linked to a reduction in risk of long-term outcomes. In a meta-analysis of hypertension, the use of ARB (13%), ACE inhibitors (10%), and calcium antagonist (11%) was associated with the greatest reduction in LV mass from baseline compared with diuretics (8%) and β-blockers (6%).[13] The choice of agent to use, however, is also based on other factors as recommended in the hypertension guidelines.[14]

Because myocardial ischemia may worsen HFpEF, its presence should be detected and, if present, treated using anti-ischemic therapies, which include β-blockers, calcium antagonists, and nitrates. Patients with evidence of myocardial ischemia could also be considered for revascularization with percutaneous coronary intervention or by coronary artery bypass graft surgery, especially if they have drug-refractory angina or angina-equivalent symptoms.

Diagnosis and treatment of obstructive sleep apnea, which has been associated with the development of diastolic dysfunction, is also important. Therapy with continuous positive airway pressure may reverse diastolic dysfunction and reduce left atrial size as measured by Doppler echocardiography, although treatment of sleep apnea has not been shown to reverse HFpEF in trials.[15]

Treatment of iron deficiency may improve symptoms and quality of life in patients with HFrEF, as demonstrated in the Fair-HF trial, which randomized 459 patients with HFrEF with evidence of iron deficiency with or without anemia to intravenous iron or placebo.[16] Whether intravenous iron is useful in HFpEF will be determined by future studies.

Obesity, diabetes mellitus, and renal dysfunction are associated with ventricular-vascular characteristics that contribute to HFpEF.[17] Optimal treatment of chronic obstructive pulmonary disease is also recommended.

It is recommended that HFpEF patients receive the pneumococcal vaccination and the annual influenza vaccination.

PHARMACOLOGIC STRATEGIES

Most drug trials have failed to improve outcomes in HFpEF (**Table 2**). This section gives an overview of pharmacologic trials and studies. Several factors may be responsible for the failure of trials to show

a benefit of specific therapies in HFpEF. These include uncertainties surrounding the pathophysiology of HFpEF, the lack of consensus in the definition and classification of HFpEF with resulting inability to clearly define the patient population, and potential use of end points or analyses that may not be ideal in HFpEF. Moreover, patients with this heterogeneous syndrome might in fact respond to different types of therapies, which would require more accurate phenotyping. For example, HFpEF patients with EF of 45% to 50% may with elevated natriuretic peptide levels behave more like patients with HFrEF, responding to renin-angiotensin-aldosterone system antagonism compared with those with EF greater than 50%.

ACE Inhibitors and ARBs

The rationale for the use of ACE inhibitors and ARBs in HFpEF is to block the neurohormonal pathways that lead to progression of HF and poor outcomes, as seen in HFrEF.[18]

There have been three key outcome trials using these agents in patients with HFpEF. The first, the Candesartan in Heart Failure Assessment of Reduction in Mortality and Morbidity (CHARM Preserved) trial,[19] randomized 3023 patients with an EF of greater than 40% to candesartan (up to 32 mg/day) or placebo. The trial showed a significant reduction in HF hospitalization after a median of 38 months of follow-up, but failed to demonstrate a reduction in cardiovascular (CV) mortality.

The second outcome trial, Perindopril for Elderly People with Chronic Heart Failure trial (PEP-CHF), randomized 850 elderly patients with EF greater than 40% and evidence of diastolic dysfunction on echocardiography to perindopril (titrated to 4 mg/day) or placebo.[20] This trial failed to demonstrate any reduction in the composite of all-cause mortality and HF hospitalization (the primary end point of the study) with perindopril. However, in a post hoc analysis, there was trend toward benefit with perindopril after a year follow-up.

In the third outcome trial, 4128 elderly patients with HF with EF greater than 45% were randomized to irbesartan or placebo (I-PRESERVE).[21] After 50 months of follow-up, irbesartan did not reduce the risk of the composite outcome of all-cause mortality and CV hospitalization.

Currently, guidelines do not recommend the use of ACE inhibitors or ARBs for HFpEF unless they are being used to treat comorbidities, such as hypertension.[6,7]

β-Blockers

β-blockers may have role in treating comorbidities in patients with HFpEF. Slowing an elevated heart

Table 2
Key outcome trials for heart failure with preserved ejection

Trial	Year	N	Ejection Fraction	Primary Outcome Hazard Ratio Hazard Ratio (95% Confidence Interval)	Comments
CHARM-PRESERVED Candesartan vs placebo	2003	3023	>40%	Composite of CV death and HF hospitalization 0.86 (0.74–1.0); $P = .051$	Significant reduction in HF hospitalization
PEP-CHF Peridropril vs placebo	2006	850	Wall motion index of <1.4 equivalent to EF 40%	All-cause mortality or unplanned HF hospitalization 0.69 (0.47–1.01); $P = .055$ at 12 months	Post hoc analysis showed a trend toward benefit with perindopril at 12 mo
I-PRESERVE Irbesartan vs placebo	2008	4128	>45%	All-cause mortality or hospitalization for CV cause 0.95 (0.86–1.05); $P = .35$	None
DIG Digoxin vs placebo	2006	988	>45%	Composite of HF hospitalization and HF mortality 0.82 (0.63–1.07); $P = .136$	Trend toward reduction in HF hospitalization
SENIORS Nebivolol vs placebo	2005	2128	>35%	All-cause mortality or hospitalization for CV cause 0.86 (0.74–0.99); $P = .039$	Cut off of EF of 35% makes it difficult to extrapolate these data to HFpEF population
TOPCAT Spironolactone vs placebo	2014	3445	>45%	Composite of death from CV causes, aborted arrest, or hospitalization for HF 0.89 (0.77–1.04); $P = .14$	HF hospitalization was reduced by 17% relative to placebo group Prespecified subgroup analysis demonstrated that patients enrolled with elevated natriuretic peptides as opposed to previous history of hospitalization had a significant reduction in primary outcome

rate can prolong LV filling time in abnormally stiff LV and also prolong coronary perfusion. Therefore, rate limitation and maintenance of atrial fibrillation with β-blockers is beneficial.[22] However, there is also a high prevalence of chronotropic incompetence in patients with HFpEF, which may already be a contributing factor to symptoms because of limited increase in cardiac output with exertion,[23–25] and in these circumstances the use of β-blocker is not recommended. The evidence base for clinical efficacy for the use of β-blocker therapy in HFpEF is inconclusive. The SENIORS trial, which randomized 2128 patients older than 70 years of age with EF ≤ 35% to placebo or nebivolol, resulted in significant reduction of all-cause

mortality and CV hospitalization after 21 months of follow-up.[26] A prespecified post hoc analysis of the trial demonstrated that the effect of nebivolol on outcomes was similar in those with preserved and impaired LVEF.[27] However, the definition of HFpEF used a low cutoff EF of greater than 35% therefore making it difficult to extrapolate these findings to most patients with HFpEF who have a higher EF. Registry data have been controversial, because the OPTMIZE-HF study did not show any benefit with β-blockers.[28] However, the COHERE registry (Carvedilol Heart Failure Registry) demonstrated that carvedilol use was associated with lower mortality and need for rehospitalization in those with EF of greater than

40%.[29] Current guidelines do not recommend the use of β-blockers solely for HFpEF, unless it is used to optimize treatment of comorbidity, such as controlling ventricular rate in atrial fibrillation or tachyarrhythmia, treating angina, or hypertension.[6,7]

Digoxin

The Digitalis Investigation Group (DIG) ancillary trial, randomized 988 patients with EF greater than 45% to digoxin or placebo.[30] After a median of 37 months of follow-up, digoxin resulted in a trend toward reduction in HF hospitalization but it did not result in a reduction in all-cause mortality, HF, or CV mortality, or the composite outcome of HF death or hospitalization. Similar to β-blockers, guidelines do not recommend the use of digoxin solely for HFpEF, unless it is used to optimize treatment of comorbidity, such as controlling ventricular rate in atrial fibrillation or tachyarrhythmia.[6,7]

Calcium Antagonists

Data regarding the use of calcium antagonist are restricted to small studies that have shown that rate-limiting calcium antagonists, such as verapamil, may lead to improved symptoms and exercise tolerance.[31] There are no outcome studies using calcium antagonists. Current guidelines do not recommend the use of calcium antagonists solely for HFpEF, unless it is used to optimize treatment of comorbidity, such as controlling ventricular rate in atrial fibrillation or tachyarrhythmia, treating angina, or hypertension.[6,7]

Aldosterone Antagonist

A potential rationale for aldosterone antagonist therapy for HFpEF comes from animal studies suggesting that aldosterone contributes to cardiac hypertrophy and fibrosis.[32] By blocking aldosterone these processes may be prevented or reversed.[33,34] The first key study using aldosterone was Aldosterone Receptor Blockade in Diastolic Heart Failure (ALDO-HF),[35] in which 422 patients were randomized to spironolactone, 25 mg per day, or placebo. After 12 months of follow-up, spironolactone was associated with improved diastolic dysfunction (assessed by e/e' ratio by Doppler echocardiography), reduced LV mass, and reduced N-terminal pro brain natriuretic peptide (NT-proBNP). However, spironolactone did not improve the coprimary outcome of peak VO_2 or for measures of quality of life.

The Treatment of Preserved Cardiac Function Heart Failure with an Aldosterone Antagonist (TOPCAT) trial[36] randomized 3445 patients with HFpEF, EF greater than 45%, to placebo or spironolactone, 45 mg per day. There was no difference in rates of the primary outcome of death from CV causes, aborted cardiac arrest, or hospitalization for HF over a mean follow-up of 3.3 years. However, HF hospitalization was significantly reduced (17% relative reduction) in patients receiving spironolactone. Of note, patients on spironolactone had double the risk of developing hyperkalemia and a higher rate of increased serum creatinine levels but a lower rate of hypokalemia compared with the placebo group. Prespecified subgroup analyses showed that patients enrolled according to elevated natriuretic peptides criteria as opposed to hospitalization for HF criteria did have a reduction in the primary outcome. However, this entry measure was highly confounded by region and post hoc analyses revealed that patients from the Americas (United States, Canada, Argentina, and Brazil) had a substantially higher event rate than those enrolled in Russia and the Republic of Georgia. Although TOPCAT did not meet its primary end point, and thus spironolactone cannot be recommended based on these results, clinicians who decide to use it in their patients with HFpEF should carefully monitor potassium and renal function.

Studies of Novel Therapies

Several key proof-of-concept studies have focused on the new paradigm of the pathophysiology of HFpEF, which targets the disrupted nitric oxide–cGMP-PKG pathway, which is associated with endothelial dysfunction caused by lack of nitric oxide availability, which is implicated in the development of concentric remodeling, increased stiffness of cardiomyocytes, and increased myocardial collagen deposition in patients with HFpEF.

One promising new agent is LCZ696, a first in class angiotensin receptor neprilysin inhibitor, which consists of a molecular complex of the ARB valsartan and the neprilysin inhibitor precursor AHU377 in a 1:1 ratio. After ingestion, the two components separate and AHU377 is converted to the active neprilysin inhibitor, LBQ377. Neprilysin degrades several vasoactive peptides including the biologically active natriuretic peptides ANP, BNP, and CNP, which in turn exert their effects by raising intracellular cGMP.

In the PARAMOUNT study, 301 patients with HFpEF were randomized to valsartan or LCZ696 and followed up for 36 weeks.[37] The primary end point of the study was a change in NT-proBNP at 12 weeks from baseline, which was significantly lower in the LCZ696 arm. At 36 weeks, left atrial volumes were reduced and New York Heart Association class was improved in the LCZ696 arm. A large outcome trial, PARAGON-HF, will assess the efficacy and safety of LCZ696 in patients with HFpEF (clinicaltrials.gov NCT01920711).

An initial small clinical study of sildenafil, a phosphodiesterase-5 inhibitor that can lead to increased levels of cGMP, in 44 patients with HFpEF (EF ≥50%) and pulmonary hypertension resulted in improved LV diastolic function, reduced pulmonary pressures, and improved right ventricular systolic function after treatment for a year.

However, these benefits where not reported in the placebo-controlled RELAX trial, which assessed the effects of sildenafil in 216 elderly patients with HFpEF without pulmonary hypertension.[38] After 24 weeks of treatment, there were no improvements in exercise capacity measured by 6-minute walk distance or on quality of life; also there were no improvements in diastolic function or LV remodeling. The lack of benefit of sildenafil in the RELAX trial could be because the patients enrolled did not have pulmonary hypertension and as suggested by very high NT-proBNP levels had advanced HF and were therefore less likely to respond to sildenafil treatment.

Another group of agents being studied are stimulators of the soluble guanylate cyclase. The latter acts as a receptor for nitric oxide. Stimulation of soluble guanylate cyclase can lead to increased activity of the cGMP-PKG pathway. The oral soluble guanylate cyclase stimulator, BAY1021189, is currently being investigated in patients with worsening HFpEF (SOCRATES-PRESERVED; clinicaltrials.gov NCT01951638).

In the SHIFT trial, heart rate reduction with ivabradine, an inhibitor of the I_f channel within cardiomyocytes of the sinoatrial node, resulted in a significant relative reduction in the primary end point of hospitalization for HF and CV mortality by 18% in patients with HFrEF, mainly driven by a reduction in HF hospitalization.[39] The use of ivabradine in patients with HFpEF is limited to a recent trial of 61 patients with HFpEF, randomized to placebo or ivabradine, 5 mg twice a day. The ivabradine arm had improved exercise capacity caused by improved LV filling pressures.[40] A larger multicenter placebo-controlled trial enrolling 400 patients will evaluate the effects of ivabradine on exercise capacity, NT-proBNP levels, and echocardiographic parameters of LV diastolic function, such as e/e' (www.clinicaltrialsregister.eu-EUCTR2012-002742-20-DE).

NONPHARMACOLOGIC STRATEGIES

Nonpharmacologic strategies for the management of HFpEF include the potential use of exercise training. In the EX-DHF-Pilot study,[41] 64 patients with HFpEF were randomized to exercise training and usual care or usual care alone. After 3 months, patients who had regular supervised exercise had an increase in peak VO_2, improved self-reported physical functioning (as assessed by the Short Form-36 health questionnaire), and improved diastolic function and reverse atrial remodeling. A larger trial of exercise training is underway.

The recent COMPASS trial showed that wireless monitoring of pulmonary arterial pressure using an implantable device was safe and resulted in reduced hospitalization in patients with HF.[42] This trial included patients with HFpEF. However, the device is currently not available for clinical use, but is potentially very promising. The results of trials of remote monitoring using such parameters as weight, heart, and blood pressure monitoring have been mixed and controversial.

SUMMARY

The management of HFpEF is challenging, requiring an accurate diagnosis. Although currently there is no convincing therapy that can prolong survival in patients with HFpEF, treatment of fluid retention and of comorbidities, such as hypertension, myocardial ischemia, and atrial fibrillation, may improve symptoms and quality of life. Spironolactone may be considered in patients with HFpEF with an elevated BNP, and if prescribed, patients require monitoring of potassium levels and renal function. Future outcome trials of HFpEF testing the efficacy of promising new agents, such as LCZ696, will have better characterization of patient phenotype to maximize the potential response to therapies.

REFERENCES

1. Bhatia RS, Tu JV, Lee DS, et al. Outcome of heart failure with preserved ejection fraction in a population-based study. N Engl J Med 2006;355(3):260–9.

2. Lam CS, Donal E, Kraigher-Krainer E, et al. Epidemiology and clinical course of heart failure with preserved ejection fraction. Eur J Heart Fail 2011; 13(1):18–28.

3. Owan TE, Hodge DO, Herges RM, et al. Trends in prevalence and outcome of heart failure with preserved ejection fraction. N Engl J Med 2006;355(3): 251–9.

4. Go AS, Mozaffarian D, Roger VL, et al, American Heart Association Statistics Committee, Stroke Statistics Subcommittee. Heart disease and stroke statistics–2014 update: a report from the American Heart Association. Circulation 2014;129(3): e28–292.

5. Chan MM, Lam CS. How do patients with heart failure with preserved ejection fraction die? Eur J Heart Fail 2013;15(6):604–13.

6. McMurray JJ, Adamopoulos S, Anker SD, et al, ESC Committee for Practice Guidelines. ESC Guidelines for the diagnosis and treatment of acute and chronic heart failure 2012: the Task Force for the Diagnosis and Treatment of Acute and Chronic Heart Failure 2012 of the European Society of Cardiology. Developed in collaboration with the Heart Failure Association (HFA) of the ESC. Eur Heart J 2012;33(14):1787–847.

7. Yancy CW, Jessup M, Bozkurt B, et al, American College of Cardiology Foundation, American Heart Association Task Force on Practice Guidlines. 2013 ACCF/AHA guideline for the management of heart failure: a report of the American College of Cardiology Foundation/American Heart Association Task Force on Practice Guidelines. J Am Coll Cardiol 2013;62(16):e147–239.

8. Jefferies JL, Bartone C, Menon S, et al. Ultrafiltration in heart failure with preserved ejection fraction: comparison with systolic heart failure patients. Circ Heart Fail 2013;6(4):733–9.

9. Ather S, Chan W, Bozkurt B, et al. Impact of noncardiac comorbidities on morbidity and mortality in a predominantly male population with heart failure and preserved versus reduced ejection fraction. J Am Coll Cardiol 2012;59(11):998–1005.

10. Beckett NS, Peters R, Fletcher AE, et al. Treatment of hypertension in patients 80 years of age or older. N Engl J Med 2008;358(18):1887–98.

11. ALLHAT Officers and Coordinators for the ALLHAT Collaborative Research Group, The Antihypertensive and Lipid-Lowering Treatment to Prevent Heart Attack Trial. Major outcomes in high-risk hypertensive patients randomized to angiotensin-converting enzyme inhibitor or calcium channel blocker vs diuretic: the Antihypertensive and Lipid-Lowering Treatment to Prevent Heart Attack Trial (ALLHAT). JAMA 2002;288(23):2981–97.

12. Wachtell K, Bella JN, Rokkedal J, et al. Change in diastolic left ventricular filling after one year of antihypertensive treatment: the Losartan Intervention For Endpoint Reduction in Hypertension (LIFE) Study. Circulation 2002;105(9):1071–6.

13. Klingbeil AU, Schneider M, Martus P, et al. A meta-analysis of the effects of treatment on left ventricular mass in essential hypertension. Am J Med 2003;115(1):41–6.

14. James PA, Oparil S, Carter BL, et al. 2014 evidence-based guideline for the management of high blood pressure in adults: report from the panel members appointed to the Eighth Joint National Committee (JNC 8). JAMA 2014;311(5):507–20.

15. Butt M, Dwivedi G, Shantsila A, et al. Left ventricular systolic and diastolic function in obstructive sleep apnea: impact of continuous positive airway pressure therapy. Circ Heart Fail 2012;5(2):226–33.

16. Anker SD, Comin Colet J, Filippatos G, et al. Ferric carboxymaltose in patients with heart failure and iron deficiency. N Engl J Med 2009;361(25):2436–48.

17. Mohammed SF, Borlaug BA, Roger VL, et al. Comorbidity and ventricular and vascular structure and function in heart failure with preserved ejection fraction: a community-based study. Circ Heart Fail 2012;5(6):710–9.

18. Benedict CR, Johnstone DE, Weiner DH, et al. Relation of neurohumoral activation to clinical variables and degree of ventricular dysfunction: a report from the Registry of Studies of Left Ventricular Dysfunction. SOLVD Investigators. J Am Coll Cardiol 1994;23(6):1410–20.

19. Yusuf S, Pfeffer MA, Swedberg K, et al, CHARM Investigators and Committees. Effects of candesartan in patients with chronic heart failure and preserved left-ventricular ejection fraction: the CHARM-PRESERVED Trial. Lancet 2003;362(9386):777–81.

20. Cleland JG, Tendera M, Adamus J, et al. The perindopril in elderly people with chronic heart failure (PEP-CHF) study. Eur Heart J 2006;27(19):2338–45.

21. Massie BM, Carson PE, McMurray JJ, et al. Irbesartan in patients with heart failure and preserved ejection fraction. N Engl J Med 2008;359(23):2456–67.

22. Bonow RO, Udelson JE. Left ventricular diastolic dysfunction as a cause of congestive heart failure. Mechanisms and management. Ann Intern Med 1992;117(6):502–10.

23. Borlaug BA, Olson TP, Lam CS, et al. Global cardiovascular reserve dysfunction in heart failure with preserved ejection fraction. J Am Coll Cardiol 2010;56(11):845–54.

24. Phan TT, Abozguia K, Nallur Shivu G, et al. Heart failure with preserved ejection fraction is characterized by dynamic impairment of active relaxation and contraction of the left ventricle on exercise and associated with myocardial energy deficiency. J Am Coll Cardiol 2009;54(5):402–9.

25. Phan TT, Shivu GN, Abozguia K, et al. Impaired heart rate recovery and chronotropic incompetence in patients with heart failure with preserved ejection fraction. Circ Heart Fail 2010;3(1):29–34.

26. Flather MD, Shibata MC, Coats AJ, et al. Randomized trial to determine the effect of nebivolol on mortality and cardiovascular hospital admission in elderly patients with heart failure (SENIORS). Eur Heart J 2005;26(3):215–25.

27. van Veldhuisen DJ, Cohen-Solal A, Bohm M, et al. Beta-blockade with nebivolol in elderly heart failure patients with impaired and preserved left ventricular ejection fraction: data from SENIORS (Study of Effects of Nebivolol Intervention on Outcomes and Rehospitalization in Seniors With Heart Failure). J Am Coll Cardiol 2009;53(23):2150–8.

28. Hernandez AF, Hammill BG, O'Connor CM, et al. Clinical effectiveness of beta-blockers in heart failure: findings from the OPTIMIZE-HF (Organized Program to Initiate Lifesaving Treatment in Hospitalized Patients with Heart Failure) registry. J Am Coll Cardiol 2009;53(2):184–92.

29. Massie BM, Nelson JJ, Lukas MA, et al. Comparison of outcomes and usefulness of carvedilol across a spectrum of left ventricular ejection fractions in patients with heart failure in clinical practice. Am J Cardiol 2007;99(9):1263–8.

30. Ahmed A, Rich MW, Fleg JL, et al. Effects of digoxin on morbidity and mortality in diastolic heart failure: the ancillary digitalis investigation group trial. Circulation 2006;114(5):397–403.

31. Setaro JF, Zaret BL, Schulman DS, et al. Usefulness of verapamil for congestive heart failure associated with abnormal left ventricular diastolic filling and normal left ventricular systolic performance. Am J Cardiol 1990;66(12):981–6.

32. Lijnen P, Petrov V. Induction of cardiac fibrosis by aldosterone. J Mol Cell Cardiol 2000;32(6):865–79.

33. Lacolley P, Safar ME, Lucet B, et al. Prevention of aortic and cardiac fibrosis by spironolactone in old normotensive rats. J Am Coll Cardiol 2001;37(2):662–7.

34. Weber KT, Brilla CG. Pathological hypertrophy and cardiac interstitium. Fibrosis and renin-angiotensin-aldosterone system. Circulation 1991;83(6):1849–65.

35. Edelmann F, Wachter R, Schmidt AG, et al. Effect of spironolactone on diastolic function and exercise capacity in patients with heart failure with preserved ejection fraction: the Aldo-DHF randomized controlled trial. JAMA 2013;309(8):781–91.

36. Pitt B, Pfeffer MA, Assmann SF, et al. Spironolactone for heart failure with preserved ejection fraction. N Engl J Med 2014;370(15):1383–92.

37. Solomon SD, Zile M, Pieske B, et al. Prospective comparison of AwARBoMOhfwpefl. The angiotensin receptor neprilysin inhibitor LCZ696 in heart failure with preserved ejection fraction: a phase 2 double-blind randomised controlled trial. Lancet 2012; 380(9851):1387–95.

38. Redfield MM, Chen HH, Borlaug BA, et al. Effect of phosphodiesterase-5 inhibition on exercise capacity and clinical status in heart failure with preserved ejection fraction: a randomized clinical trial. JAMA 2013;309(12):1268–77.

39. Swedberg K, Komajda M, Bohm M, et al. Ivabradine and outcomes in chronic heart failure (SHIFT): a randomised placebo-controlled study. Lancet 2010; 376(9744):875–85.

40. Kosmala W, Holland DJ, Rojek A, et al. Effect of If-channel inhibition on hemodynamic status and exercise tolerance in heart failure with preserved ejection fraction: a randomized trial. J Am Coll Cardiol 2013; 62(15):1330–8.

41. Edelmann F, Gelbrich G, Dungen HD, et al. Exercise training improves exercise capacity and diastolic function in patients with heart failure with preserved ejection fraction: results of the Ex-DHF (Exercise training in Diastolic Heart Failure) pilot study. J Am Coll Cardiol 2011;58(17):1780–91.

42. Abraham WT, Adamson PB, Bourge RC, et al. Wireless pulmonary artery haemodynamic monitoring in chronic heart failure: a randomised controlled trial. Lancet 2011;377(9766):658–66.

Potential Applications of Pharmacogenomics to Heart Failure Therapies

Kishan S. Parikh, MD[a],*, Tariq Ahmad, MD, MPH[a,b],
Mona Fiuzat, PharmD[a,b]

KEYWORDS

- Pharmacogenomics • Pharmacogenetics • Heart failure • Personalized medicine

KEY POINTS

- Pharmacogenomics refers to polymorphisms within the genome that may modify the individual response to treatment.
- Anywhere between 20% and 95% of the variability of a drug's response can be caused by genetic effects.
- Traditional heart failure management based on large, randomized trials and pharmacogenomics can form a complementary relationship to outline specific therapeutic options among a predefined patient population.
- Possible uses for pharmacogenomics in heart failure range from specific disease conditions, including pulmonary hypertension (PH), to optimization of well-established therapies, such as β-blockers and implantable cardiac defibrillators.
- Although the field is growing rapidly, pharmacogenomics in heart failure is still quite young and not quite ready for clinical application at the moment.

BACKGROUND

Pharmacogenomics refers to polymorphisms within the genome that may modify an individual response to treatment, and the field has evolved alongside modern medicine. Although not equipped with the genetic knowledge of modern day, Sir William Osler[1] observed in 1892 that decompensation of patients with heart failure (HF) occurs at different rates, bringing attention to the heterogeneity with which the syndrome manifests.[1,2] A few decades later, in 1923, the English physiologist Archibald Garrod[3] noted that genetic variation may lead to variability in accumulation of both endogenous and exogenous products, including drugs.[3] With the help of the human genome project and genome-wide association studies (GWAS) over the last few decades, these basic concepts have propelled significant advances in therapies for oncology and infectious disease and have brought a better understanding of how best to dose cardiac therapeutics, such as antiplatelet agents and warfarin. Indeed, it is estimated that anywhere between 20% and 95% of the variability of a drug's response can be caused by genetic effects.[4]

On first glance, the idea of personalized medicine stands in stark contrast to the modern management of HF, which has been molded by large, randomized clinical trials comparing the effects of rival therapies on a single, phenotypically similar population.[5] Pharmacogenomics instead explores one drug's varying effects on different patient genotypes. However, the overall objectives of both

Disclosures: none.
[a] Division of Cardiology, Duke University Medical Center, 3428, Durham, NC 27710, USA; [b] Duke Clinical Research Institute, DUMC Box 3356, Durham, NC 27710, USA
* Corresponding author.
E-mail address: kishan.parikh@duke.edu

are complementary and together can effectively outline an optimal algorithm for therapy (including drug, dose, duration, safety, and efficacy) in a pre-defined HF population. The utility of pharmacogenomics in HF will likely also increase, as drug regimens become more complex and new pharmacologic interactions and dosing considerations surface.

A better understanding of genomic variation's contribution to drug response can impact 4 arenas in HF: (1) identification of patients most likely to receive benefit from therapy, (2) risk stratify patients for risk of adverse events, (3) optimize dosing of drugs, and (4) steer future clinical trial design and drug development (**Fig. 1**).[4] Although the body of literature for pharmacogenomics of HF therapies is quite young, the field has already made initial significant advances and shows great promise.[6,7] In this review, the authors explore potential applications of pharmacogenomics in patients with HF in the context of these categories.

THE UNMET NEED FOR OPTIMIZATION OF HF DRUG REGIMEN

HF is a public health problem of massive proportions in both developed and developing countries: In the United States alone, more than 5 million patients are estimated to have HF, more than 1 million hospitalizations and 270,000 deaths result annually from HF, and disease management accounts for more than $30 billion in total costs per annum.[8] However, evidence-based therapies, such as β-blockers and renin-angiotensin-aldosterone system (RAAS) inhibitors, that can significantly improve outcomes in HF continue to

be used at doses far less than their thresholds for therapeutic efficacy. In part, this practice is a result of significant interpatient variation in what defines an optimized medical regimen, likely a function of genetic variation, patient behavior, and disease state.

Achieving an optimized medical regimen is critical to establish the best potential for recovery of ventricular function and is also becoming more complex as more options arise with new drugs and therapeutic combinations for different patient populations.[9] Fine-tuning the correct dose and balance of medications for patients can be challenging and traditionally has depended on several components, including patient tolerance, cost, compliance, and comorbid conditions. Frequently, several medications with proven mortality benefit in HF must be compared with each other during titration and selected in order of efficacy for initiation/dose increase. Preference given to one medication relies in part on the physician's gestalt because it cannot be known how well the theoretic benefit based on prior studies matches the patients' response to the drug. With an understanding of variability in drug response, whether a patient is more likely to have an adverse effect or have the desired response can be known before starting the drug. β-blockers, aldosterone antagonists, and angiotensin-converting enzyme inhibitors are among the most commonly used drugs in HF and have been examined for a genetic basis to explain patients' heterogeneous responses. In a short period of time, significant advances in pharmacogenomics have laid the groundwork for significantly improving HF management.

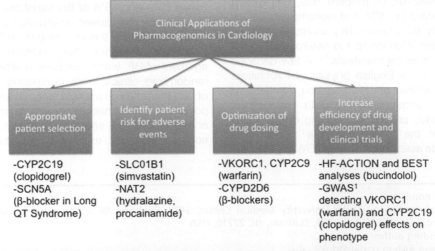

Fig. 1. Four broad arenas for potential pharmacogenomic use in cardiology have been established but require further exploration. [1] GWAS, genome-wide association study.

β-Blockers

β-blockers significantly reduce morbidity and mortality in patients with HF and continue to be a cornerstone of chronic HF therapy.[10–14] Despite the supporting data for this class of drugs, its effects and tolerability vary significantly across a phenotypically diverse HF population. The $β_1$-adrenergic receptor (AR) has been examined for genetic variation over the past decade; in particular, the position 389 Arg/Gly polymorphism has been studied with greatest interest. This polymorphism exists because of a nucleotide 1165 C(Arg) → G(Gly) transversion that alters signaling in multiple pathways contributing to HF. The $β_1$-Arg-389 allele, reported to be present in 62% of blacks and 73% of non-blacks, may confer a survival benefit in patients with HF taking the β-blocker bucindolol, whereas patients with the $β_1$-Gly-389 allele have been shown to have no response to bucindolol compared with placebo. A large randomized trial of β-blockers in HF, the β-Blocker Evaluation of Survival Trial, also included a 1040-patient DNA substudy based on the $β_1$ AR genotype and found similar results between $β_1$ 389 Arg homozygotes and $β_1$ 389 AR Gly carriers.[15] In support that this polymorphism truly affects the drug response and not natural disease progression of HF, patients receiving placebo with both genotypes did not have any significant difference in morbidity and mortality. Significant gene-dose interactions have also been discovered: a DNA analysis from the Participants in Heart Failure: A Controlled Trial Investigating Outcomes of Exercise Training showed that Arg homozygotes had a 2-fold increase in the risk of death if taking low-dose β-blockers instead of high-dose β-blockers (**Fig. 2**).[16] This risk was not observed in Gly carriers.

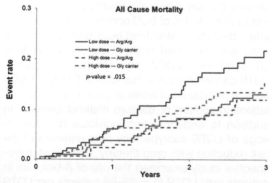

Fig. 2. Adjusted Kaplan-Meier curves for all-cause mortality by dose of β-blocker and $β_1$-Arg-389 genotype. (*From* Fiuzat M, Neely ML, Starr AZ, et al. Association between adrenergic receptor genotypes and beta-blocker dose in heart failure patients: analysis from the HF-ACTION DNA substudy. Eur J Heart Fail 2013;15:258–66; with permission.)

However, other randomized trials have tested the impact of the $β_1$ 389 AR Arg/Gly polymorphism on mortality and hospitalizations in patients taking long-acting metoprolol and carvedilol.[12,17] No change in mortality, hospitalizations, or drug effect (metoprolol CR/XL, metoprolol succinate, and carvedilol) was found between both groups of patients.

The reason for these conflicting findings may be related to bucindolol's unique ability to inactivate constitutively active $β_1$ ARs or its enhanced sympatholytic properties compared with other β-blockers.[9,15,18–21] The synergistic relationship of the $β_1$ 389 AR Arg polymorphism with another polymorphism, $α_{2C}$ Del322–325, may also explain these contradictory findings, especially in black patients (**Fig. 3**).[22] Decreased function of the $α_{2C}$ receptor (allele frequency of 41.1% in blacks vs 3.8% in whites) increases effective circulating norepinephrine levels; when present with the $β_1$ 389 AR Arg polymorphism, the risk for HF in blacks increases by 10-fold.[22] By establishing an HF phenotype, the presence or absence of these polymorphisms could guide early HF management and therapy.

Genetic testing for the response to β-blocker therapy in HF is not yet ready for common clinical practice but shows promise in helping optimize HF regimens. Further clinical studies are needed to better elucidate the $β_1$ AR genotypes and their impact on β-blockade.

RAAS

Polymorphisms in the RAAS have also been investigated. Similar to β-blockers, drugs targeting the RAAS have been shown to produce a variable therapeutic response with a genetic basis. However, until recently, much of the studies exploring genes of interest in HF had come from mostly white patient populations, such as the Genetic Risk Assessment of Cardiac Events (GRACE) study.[23] A DNA substudy called the Genetic Risk Assessment of Heart Failure in African Americans (GRAHF) was conducted to begin addressing this inadequacy using data from the African American Heart Failure Trial (AHeFT). AHeFT compared the combination of isosorbide dinitrate and hydralazine with placebo in patients already receiving standard HF therapy.[24] In GRAHF, the aldosterone synthase gene (*CYP11B2*) position 344 T/C polymorphism was investigated, as it has been shown that the −344C allele binds to the steroidogenic transcription factor involved in the aldosterone synthesis pathway with 4 times greater affinity than the 344T allele and is associated with greater aldosterone production.[24–26] Not only was

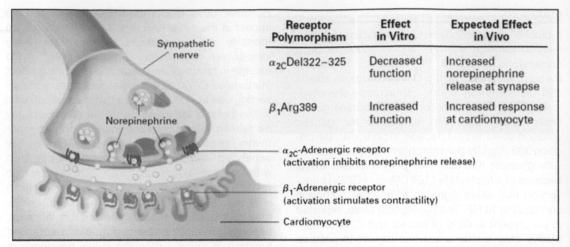

Receptor Polymorphism	Effect in Vitro	Expected Effect in Vivo
α_{2C}Del322–325	Decreased function	Increased norepinephrine release at synapse
β_1Arg389	Increased function	Increased response at cardiomyocyte

α_{2C}-Adrenergic receptor (activation inhibits norepinephrine release)

β_1-Adrenergic receptor (activation stimulates contractility)

Cardiomyocyte

Fig. 3. Polymorphisms affecting norepinephrine signaling have been shown to significantly affect response to β-blocker therapy. (*From* Small KM, Wagoner LE, Levin AM, et al. Synergistic polymorphisms of beta1- and alpha2C-adrenergic receptors and the risk of congestive heart failure. N Engl J Med 2002;347:1135–42; with permission.)

freedom from hospitalization significantly better in TT homozygotes versus heterozygotes and CC homozygotes but this group of patients also experienced the greatest improvement in quality of life with isosorbide and hydralazine treatment. Furthermore, the GRAHF substudy also demonstrated a significant difference in prevalence of TT homozygosity by race. The −344 TT genotype was present in approximately twice as many blacks as in a white patient cohort of the GRACE study (62% vs 30%). Given the low-renin hypertension (increased aldosterone-to-renin ratio) and associated cardiomyopathy that is more common in blacks, these findings may contain important and practical prognostic as well as therapeutic information for pharmacologic consideration.

PREVENTION OF SUDDEN CARDIAC DEATH

Pharmacogenomics also has a potential use for nondrug therapy in HF. Sudden cardiac death (SCD) prevalence continues to increase despite an overall decrease in cardiovascular mortality, largely because of an increasing cohort of patients living with HF and coronary artery disease and an inability to accurately predict who will have SCD.[27] Implantable cardiac defibrillators (ICDs) for both primary and secondary prevention of SCD reduce mortality in HF and have been shown to be cost-effective[28]; but as the HF population grows in size and age, increasing attention is shifting toward appropriate patient selection. It is estimated that only 1 in 11 patients who receive prophylactic ICD therapy will require an appropriate shock.[29,30] Several other reasons to carefully

consider ICD placement include limited financial resources, implantation and device complications, and inappropriate shocks. In addition, those patients at highest risk for SCD may not be obviously highlighted by traditional risk factors alone. Age, prior myocardial infarction, low ejection fraction, and prior history of aborted SCD are powerful predictors of SCD; but reliance on these characteristics alone has limitations. For example, only one-third of the patients who experience SCD actually have low ejection fraction.[31] The ability to assess the individual, refined risk for SCD would, therefore, certainly be a useful tool.

Several polymorphisms contribute to the initiation and propagation of life-threatening arrhythmias, but the overall inheritance of SCD (both with and without structural heart disease) remains poorly defined. Approximately 5% of SCD occurs without coronary artery disease or structural heart disease, and the most well described of these conditions are long QT syndrome (LQTS) and Brugada syndrome. LQTS can result from either loss-of-function mutations in potassium channel or gain-of-function mutations in sodium or calcium channel genes.[32] In addition to understanding individual risk, knowledge of LQTS subtype may help understand the risk reduction with drug therapy. One small, retrospective study examined the use of β-blockers in patients with LQTS (n = 28–69 patients per LQTS subtype).[33] LQT1 and LQT2 (potassium channel mutations) were shown to have a significantly reduced risk for SCD if on β-blocker therapy, but patients with LQT3 (SCN5A mutation in calcium channel) show no response to β-blockade. In addition to heritable syndromes, SCD occurring after myocardial infarction also likely has a familial component.[34] Four retrospective, case-control studies have shown that independent of a family history of myocardial infarction, the presence of SCD in a first-degree relative conferred a 1.6- to 2.7-fold risk of ventricular arrhythmia.[35–38] The genetic basis and, therefore, a potential targeted therapeutic approach are yet to be elucidated in these patients. To this end, a large, prospective trial called the Prospective Observational Study of Implantable Cardioverter Defibrillators in Primary Prevention of Sudden Cardiac Death is currently underway with a target enrollment of 1200 patients with a history of myocardial infarction and ejection fraction less than 30% in which genomic analysis will be performed along with structural phenotyping. Ultimately, several polymorphisms found to be associated with specific arrhythmogenic syndromes could be assembled in a panel that could be clinically tested as well as used in translational research for novel therapeutics.

PULMONARY ARTERIAL HYPERTENSION

Pulmonary hypertension (PH) is broadly defined as a mean pulmonary arterial pressure of 25 mm Hg or more at rest. The natural progression of the disease is right HF, with an estimated 1-year mortality of 10% to 15%,[39] although, before modern therapy, the estimated median survival was a dismal 2.8 years.[40,41] To further characterize the disease, the World Health Organization (WHO) has divided subtypes of the disease into 5 groups. WHO group 1, pulmonary arterial hypertension (PAH), can be idiopathic, heritable, or associated with connective tissue disease and is associated with elevated pulmonary vascular resistance because of the progressive proliferation and fibrotic changes to the small pulmonary arteries. Although a rare disease with a prevalence of approximately 10.0 million people in the United States, PAH is becoming increasingly appreciated; certain therapies approved in group 1 PH may work for groups 2 to 5. Four classes of drugs are currently approved for PAH: prostacyclin analogues, endothelin receptor antagonists, phosphodiesterase type 5 inhibitors, and soluble guanylate cyclase stimulators. Because of the phenotypic variability of the disease, limited drug options, and potential for significant adverse reactions (eg, worsening HF), PH would be an ideal fit for the application of pharmacogenomics.[42]

When familial, PAH transmission is usually autosomal dominant with reduced penetrance.[40] The gene BMPR2 codes for a type II receptor membrane of the transforming growth factor-β family, and more than 300 mutations have been associated with 80%

of familial PAH.[42,43] It is estimated that, in patients without a known family history of PAH, 20% have a germ-line mutation.[44] Genes including BMP-specific SMADs, particularly SMAD9, and KCNK3 (hypoxia-sensitive potassium channel), have also recently been identified as a possible mechanistic cause of heritable as well as idiopathic PAH in certain patients.[40] Not only has this progress been remarkable over the past decade but genetic testing and counseling to patients has also made strides. For example, a recent study of 53 families with BMPR2-related PAH showed that genetic anticipation, a previously accepted characteristic of the disease, is likely not valid in PAH.[45] Finally, clinical development of PAH therapeutics has, in part, been slowed by small sample sizes (compared with trials for drugs in other more common disease states). A pharmacogenomic application to PAH clinical trial design could have a great benefit in this aspect. By selecting appropriate subjects for testing, the use of GWAS to investigate the drug response in various diseases has shown extremely encouraging results with large odds ratios.[46] Early phase PAH clinical trials would have both increased efficiency and decreased cost with a more selective targeted subject.

Therefore, exciting potential areas of pharmacogenomics research over the next decade include identifying new targets for PAH treatment, assessing the impact of earlier treatment in patients identified through genetic testing, and exploring the utility of high-throughput techniques to identify serial progression of molecular markers in a given patient on treatment.

BRINGING THEORY INTO REALITY

As described previously, the major barriers to increasing the clinical availability of pharmacogenomics in HF include concerns about the cost-effectiveness of testing; lack of definitive data from large, prospectively designed trials; lack of integrative software to be used with an electronic medical record (EMR); and a delay in and relatively less knowledge of pharmacogenomics among health care practitioners.[47,48] Aside from the obvious need for prospective clinical trials, one potential solution to address several of these concerns is the preemptive testing of patients.[49] If several experienced, high-volume laboratories construct a genomic profile for a panel of loci in an individual patient and at a reasonable cost, then the needed information would be available for clinical use as part of the usual medical record. The Clinical Pharmacogenetics Implementation Consortium, established in 2009, has already begun creating guidelines for individual drugs to begin this effort.

Early studies at the National Institutes of Health Clinical Center investigating the impact of clinician education and EMR support seem promising and resulted in significant increases in pharmacogenomics testing of patients.[47] In a similar vein, Dewey and colleagues[50] recently reported the results of a small pilot study in which subjects had preemptive whole-genome sequencing and genetic counseling. Genomic variants, accuracy, ease of software use, and burden of clinical follow-up were critically explored. Using the online tool Pharmacogenomics Knowledge Base, drug response profiles were created for each patient. Each patient carried between 3 and 10 genetic variants associated with drug response supported by evidence level 1B or higher.[50] Finally, 11 of 12 patients carried at least one genetic variant associated with a clinical guideline recommendation for dosing change for the drugs simvastatin, warfarin,

clopidogrel, thiopurine, and codeine. A panel such as this created specifically for patients with HF who are often on lifetime therapies, with frequent dose readjustments, could be an extremely useful tool.

Finally, the investigation of HF therapeutics itself also needs increased incorporation of pharmacogenomics. Either by using a hypothesis-free approach via GWAS or testing individual candidate genes, pharmacogenomics can optimize drug development efficiency and improve the pharmacologic safety profile as postulated by Bristow[51] and others. If subjects are appropriately identified in early phase trials, the degrees of drug response can be assessed and ultimately lead to more specific stratification of appropriate target patient populations. Indeed, the benefits of pharmacogenomics-driven clinical trials seem evident in all stages of investigation (**Table 1**).[52]

Table 1
Advantages of using pharmacogenetics in various phases of clinical drug testing

Phase	Traditional Clinical Trial	Pharmacogenetics-Driven Clinical Trial
Phase I	Small group of healthy participants Designed to evaluate the safety of the new treatment	Pharmacogenetics could enable the predication of drug levels and adverse effects from known predictors of varied metabolism.
Phase II	Larger group of participants than phase I trial Designed to test the efficacy of the new treatment	From an SNP profile, patients' responsive to the drug could be differentiated from those who show no effect or even adverse events. Instead of the drug being discarded, this profiling could be used to select patients for larger phase III studies. SNP profiling of drug-response groups might identify genes contributing to heterogeneous forms of the disease and lead to the discovery of new medicines and additional targets
Phase III	Traditionally, hundreds or thousands of participants Can take several years Designed to assess adverse effects or overall lack of efficacy in population Drug approved for general use once trial is completed	Pathways determined in phase II trials are tested, and the underlying genetic variants are identified. Pharmacogenetics might allow for smaller and, therefore, more efficient phase III trials whereby treatments, dosages, or both can be stratified according to the patients' underlying genetic profile.
Phase IV	Postmarketing trials in which feedback from medical practitioners is used to evaluate the long-term safety of the treatment Designed to determine rare adverse effects in a small percentage of the population	Pharmacogenetics could be used during this phase to identify SNP markers associated with serious but rare adverse events or reduced efficacy.

Abbreviation: SNP, single nucleotide polymorphism.
From Ahmad T, Voora D, Becker RC. The pharmacogenetics of antiplatelet agents: toward personalized therapy? Nat Rev Cardiol 2011;8:562; with permission.

SUMMARY

The possible uses for pharmacogenomics in HF are expansive, ranging from specific disease conditions, including PH/right heart failure and at-risk populations for SCD, to the optimization of well-established therapies in systolic HF. Knowledge in these areas is still evolving and not quite ready for clinical application at the moment, but thus far it seems that pharmacogenomics brings potential for improved patient care, reduced adverse events, drug development, and increased cost-effectiveness in HF. Preemptive genomic testing will need to be met with caution, however. Although it continues to garner increased excitement and will likely be incorporated into clinical practice to some degree over the next 1 to 2 decades, studies like that by Dewey and colleagues[50] concurrently display the vast amount of data and clinical complexity that may be added to medical decision making. The authors approach the future of HF therapies with the addition of pharmacogenomics with cautious but strong optimism.

REFERENCES

1. Osler W. Osler: oesophagismus. Principles and practice of medicine. New York: Appleton & Co; 1892.
2. McNamara DM, Holubkov R, Janosko K, et al. Pharmacogenetic interactions between beta-blocker therapy and the angiotensin-converting enzyme deletion polymorphism in patients with congestive heart failure. Circulation 2001;103:1644–8.
3. Garrod AE. Inborn errors of metabolism. 2nd Edition. London: Oxford Univ Press; 1923.
4. Charlab R, Zhang L. Pharmacogenomics: historical perspective and current status. Methods Mol Biol 2013;1015:3–22.
5. Cappola TP, Dorn GW. Clinical considerations of heritable factors in common heart failure. Circ Cardiovasc Genet 2011;4:701–9.
6. Talameh JA, Lanfear DE. Pharmacogenetics in chronic heart failure: new developments and current challenges. Curr Heart Fail Rep 2012;9:23–32.
7. Ahmad T, O'Connor CM. Therapeutic implications of biomarkers in chronic heart failure. Clin Pharmacol Ther 2013;94:468–79.
8. Schocken DD, Benjamin EJ, Fonarow GC, et al. Prevention of heart failure: a scientific statement from the American Heart Association Councils on Epidemiology and Prevention, Clinical Cardiology, Cardiovascular Nursing, and High Blood Pressure research; Quality of Care and Outcomes Research Interdisciplinary Working Group; and Functional Genomics and Translational Biology Interdisciplinary Working Group. Circulation 2008;117:2544–65.
9. Fiuzat M, O'Connor CM, Gueyffier F, et al. Biomarker-guided therapies in heart failure: a forum for unified strategies. J Card Fail 2013;19:592–9.
10. Packer M, Coats AJS, Fowler MB, et al. Effect of carvedilol on survival in severe chronic heart failure. N Engl J Med 2001;344:1651–8.
11. Packer M, Bristow M, Cohn J, et al. The effect of carvedilol on morbidity and mortality in patients with chronic heart failure. N Engl J Med 1996;334:1349.
12. Group MH. Effect of metoprolol CR/XL in chronic heart failure: metoprolol CR/XL randomized intervention trial in congestive heart failure (MERIT-HF). Lancet 1999;353:2001.
13. Drummond GA, Squire IB. The cardiac insufficiency bisoprolol study II. Lancet 1999;353(9161):1361.
14. Flather MD, Shibata MC, Coats AJS, et al. Randomized trial to determine the effect of nebivolol on mortality and cardiovascular hospital admission in elderly patients with heart failure (SENIORS). Eur Heart J 2005;26:215–25.
15. Liggett SB, Mialet-Perez J, Thaneemit-Chen S, et al. A polymorphism within a conserved beta1-adrenergic receptor motif alters cardiac function and beta-blocker response in human heart failure. Proc Natl Acad Sci U S A 2006;103:11288–93.
16. Fiuzat M, Neely ML, Starr AZ, et al. Association between adrenergic receptor genotypes and beta-blocker dose in heart failure patients: analysis from the HF-ACTION DNA substudy. Eur J Heart Fail 2013;15:258–66.
17. Perez JM, Rathz DA, Petrashevskaya NN, et al. Beta 1-adrenergic receptor polymorphisms confer differential function and predisposition to heart failure. Nat Med 2003;9:1300–5.
18. Domanski MJ, Krause-Steinrauf H, Massie BM, et al. A comparative analysis of the results from 4 trials of β-blocker therapy for heart failure: BEST, CIBIS-II, MERIT-HF, and COPERNICUS. J Card Fail 2003;9:354–63.
19. Walsh R, Farmer R, Kelly M, et al. Human myocardial b1389 Arg/Arg adrenergic receptors exhibit a propensity for constitutively active, high affinity agonist binding and are selectively inactivated by bucindolol. J Card Fail 2008;14:S8.
20. Bristow MR, Krause-Steinrauf H, Nuzzo R, et al. Effect of baseline or changes in adrenergic activity on clinical outcomes in the beta-blocker evaluation of survival trial. Circulation 2004;110:1437–42.
21. White HL, de Boer RA, Maqbool A, et al. An evaluation of the beta-1 adrenergic receptor Arg389Gly polymorphism in individuals with heart failure: a MERIT-HF sub-study. Eur J Heart Fail 2003;5:463–8.
22. Small KM, Wagoner LE, Levin AM, et al. Synergistic polymorphisms of beta1- and alpha2C-adrenergic receptors and the risk of congestive heart failure. N Engl J Med 2002;347:1135–42.

23. McNamara DM, Holubkov R, Postava L, et al. Pharmacogenetic interactions between angiotensin-converting enzyme inhibitor therapy and the angiotensin-converting enzyme deletion polymorphism in patients with congestive heart failure. J Am Coll Cardiol 2004;44:2019–26.

24. McNamara DM, Tam SW, Sabolinski ML, et al. Aldosterone synthase promoter polymorphism predicts outcome in African Americans with heart failure: results from the A-HeFT trial. J Am Coll Cardiol 2006;48:1277–82.

25. Brand E, Chatelain N, Mulatero P, et al. Structural analysis and evaluation of the aldosterone synthase gene in hypertension. Hypertension 1998; 32:198–204.

26. White PC, Slutsker L. Haplotype analysis of CYP11B2. Endocr Res 1995;21:437–42.

27. Darbar D. Genomics, heart failure and sudden cardiac death. Heart Fail Rev 2010;15:229–38.

28. Sanders GD, Kong MH, Al-Khatib SM, et al. Cost-effectiveness of implantable cardioverter defibrillators in patients >or=65 years of age. Am Heart J 2010;160:122–31.

29. Huikuri HV, Castellanos A, Myerburg RJ. Sudden death due to cardiac arrhythmias. N Engl J Med 2001;345:1473–82.

30. Tung R, Zimetbaum P, Josephson ME. Critical appraisal of implantable cardioverter-defibrillator therapy for the prevention of sudden cardiac death. J Am Coll Cardiol 2008;52:1111–21.

31. Zipes DP, Wellens HJ. Sudden cardiac death. Circulation 1998;98:2334–51.

32. Noseworthy PA, Newton-Cheh C. Genetic determinants of sudden cardiac death. Circulation 2008; 118:1854–63.

33. Moss AJ, Zareba W, Hall WJ, et al. Effectiveness and limitations of β-Blocker therapy in congenital long-QT syndrome. Circulation 2000;101(6):616–23.

34. Frangiskakis JM, London B. Targeting device therapy: genomics of sudden death. Heart Fail Clin 2010;6:93–100.

35. Friedlander Y, Siscovick DS, Weinmann S, et al. Family history as a risk factor for primary cardiac arrest. Circulation 1998;97:155–60.

36. Jouven X, Desnos M, Guerot C, et al. Predicting sudden death in the population: the Paris prospective study I. Circulation 1999;99:1978–83.

37. Kaikkonen KS, Kortelainen ML, Linna E, et al. Family history and the risk of sudden cardiac death as a manifestation of an acute coronary event. Circulation 2006;114:1462–7.

38. Dekker LRC, Bezzina CR, Henriques JPS, et al. Familial sudden death is an important risk factor for primary ventricular fibrillation: a case-control study in acute myocardial infarction patients. Circulation 2006;114:1140–5.

39. Benza RL, Miller DP, Gomberg-Maitland M, et al. Predicting survival in pulmonary arterial hypertension: insights from the registry to evaluate early and long-term pulmonary arterial hypertension disease management (REVEAL). Circulation 2010; 122:164–72.

40. Ma L, Roman-Campos D, Austin ED, et al. A novel channelopathy in pulmonary arterial hypertension. N Engl J Med 2013;369:351–61.

41. D'Alonzo GE, Barst RJ, Ayres SM, et al. Survival in patients with primary pulmonary hypertension. Results from a national prospective registry. Ann Intern Med 1991;115:343–9.

42. Duarte JD, Hanson RL, Machado RF. Pharmacologic treatments for pulmonary hypertension: exploring pharmacogenomics. Future Cardiol 2013;9:335–49.

43. Soubrier F, Chung WK, Machado R, et al. Genetics and genomics of pulmonary arterial hypertension. J Am Coll Cardiol 2013;62:D13–21.

44. Koehler R, Grünig E, Pauciulo MW, et al. Low frequency of BMPR2 mutations in a German cohort of patients with sporadic idiopathic pulmonary arterial hypertension. J Med Genet 2004;41:e127.

45. Larkin EK, Newman JH, Austin ED, et al. Longitudinal analysis casts doubt on the presence of genetic anticipation in heritable pulmonary arterial hypertension. Am J Respir Crit Care Med 2012;186: 892–6.

46. Harper AR, Topol EJ. Pharmacogenomics in clinical practice and drug development. Nat Biotechnol 2012;30:1117–24.

47. Goldspiel BR, Flegel WA, Dipatrizio G, et al. Integrating pharmacogenetic information and clinical decision support into the electronic health record. J Am Med Inform Assoc 2013;21(3):522–8. http://dx.doi.org/10.1136/amiajnl-2013-001873.

48. Roden DM, Wilke RA, Kroemer HK, et al. Pharmacogenomics: the genetics of variable drug responses. Circulation 2011;123:1661–70.

49. Relling MV, Klein TE. CPIC: clinical pharmacogenetics implementation consortium of the pharmacogenomics research network. Clin Pharmacol Ther 2011;89:464–7.

50. Dewey FE, Grove ME, Pan C, et al. Clinical interpretation and implications of whole-genome sequencing. JAMA 2014;311:1017–9.

51. Bristow MR. Pharmacogenetic targeting of drugs for heart failure. Pharmacol Ther 2012;134:107–15.

52. Ahmad T, Voora D, Becker RC. The pharmacogenetics of antiplatelet agents: towards personalized therapy? Nat Rev Cardiol 2011;8:560–71.

Potential Roles of Vaptans in Heart Failure

Experience from Clinical Trials and Considerations for Optimizing Therapy in Target Patients

Tess E. Lin, PharmD[a], Kirkwood F. Adams Jr, MD[b],
J. Herbert Patterson, PharmD[a],*

KEYWORDS

- Aquaretic • Conivaptan • Diuretic • Dyspnea • EVEREST • Hyponatremia • Tolvaptan
- Vasopressin antagonist

KEY POINTS

- The development of vasopressin antagonists ("vaptans") in the past decade has advanced the treatment of euvolemic and hypervolemic hyponatremia. As hyponatremia is a known complication in patients with heart failure (HF) and is associated with worse outcomes, vaptans have also been studied in HF.
- In patients with HF, tolvaptan reduces body weight without adversely affecting serum electrolyte concentrations, hemodynamics, or renal function.
- Post hoc analyses from clinical trials have suggested that early administration of tolvaptan may have an optimal role in targeted patients with cardiorenal syndrome, refractory diuresis, marked hyponatremia, and/or severe congestion.
- Two prospective studies are ongoing to evaluate the hypotheses generated from analyses of previous clinical trials.

OVERVIEW

Hyponatremia is a known complication in patients with heart failure (HF), usually in the state of volume overload, or hypervolemic hyponatremia. In patients with symptomatic HF, even mildly reduced serum sodium concentrations are associated with significantly worse outcomes.[1–3] A main cause of hyponatremia is an inappropriately elevated level of plasma arginine vasopressin (AVP), which causes water retention at the collecting duct of the kidney.[4–6] Thus, AVP receptor antagonists, or "vaptans," have been developed to increase free water excretion (aquaresis) and improve serum sodium levels in patients with hyponatremia.[7–9] In the United States, 2 vaptans (conivaptan and tolvaptan) have been approved by the Food and Drug Administration (FDA) in the past decade for the treatment of euvolemic or hypervolemic hyponatremia.[10,11]

Disclosures: Dr T.E. Lin has no conflicts of interest to disclose. Dr K.F. Adams and Dr J.H. Patterson receive research support from Otsuka America Pharmaceuticals, Inc.
[a] Division of Pharmacotherapy and Experimental Therapeutics, UNC Eshelman School of Pharmacy, University of North Carolina (UNC) at Chapel Hill, CB#7355, 301 Pharmacy Lane, Chapel Hill, NC 27599-7355, USA;
[b] Division of Cardiology, UNC Heart and Vascular, University of North Carolina (UNC) at Chapel Hill, 160 Dental Circle, Chapel Hill, NC 27599-7075, USA
* Corresponding author. CB#7569, Room 3212, Kerr Hall, Chapel Hill, NC 27599-7569.
E-mail address: hpatterson@unc.edu

Heart Failure Clin 10 (2014) 607–620
http://dx.doi.org/10.1016/j.hfc.2014.07.009
1551-7136/14/$ – see front matter © 2014 Elsevier Inc. All rights reserved.

In patients with HF, vaptans have also been studied for their aquaretic effect and role in neurohormonal blockade and have consistently shown body weight reduction and increased urine output without adversely affecting serum electrolyte concentrations, hemodynamics, or renal function.[12–18] Of the vaptans, tolvaptan has been the most extensively studied among patients with HF, but it has not been approved by the FDA for the management of decompensated heart failure because of a lack of strong signal for dyspnea relief and a lack of benefit in improving all-cause mortality and morbidity.[19,20] Based on observed benefit in serum sodium correction in patients with HF in the hyponatremia trials, the use of either a V2-selective (tolvaptan) or a nonselective (conivaptan) vasopressin antagonist has been recommended as a therapeutic option in the short term to improve serum sodium concentration in hypervolemic, hyponatremic states per the 2013 American College of Cardiology Foundation/American Heart Association Guidelines for the Management of Heart Failure.[21] However, the clinical course and the impact of serum sodium correction on outcomes in this high-risk patient population remain to be studied in prospective studies. To date, only post hoc analyses of clinical trials have suggested that sodium correction in HF patients with symptomatic volume overload may be associated with favorable clinical outcomes.

For now, the optimal therapeutic niche for tolvaptan in congestive heart failure (CHF) remains to be defined. Tolvaptan's long-term safety and tolerability profile compared with loop diuretics make this aquaretic drug a potential therapeutic option for patients with decompensated HF.[18,20,22] Unfortunately, clinical trial experience with tolvaptan in HF has been complicated by inconsistency in endpoint measurements and patient populations. Complexities associated with the pathophysiology of decompensated HF and the epidemiology of this highly morbid patient population further confound clinical trial development programs and study results. Post hoc analyses have also suggested that tolvaptan may have an optimal role in targeted patients with cardiorenal syndrome, marked hyponatremia, and/or severe congestion with early administration.[17,23–26] Prospective studies are ongoing to evaluate the effects of tolvaptan in symptomatic or worsening HF patients with mild to moderate hyponatremia and/or renal insufficiency whose volume status may be difficult to manage with oral loop diuretics.[27,28] This review of the clinical trial experience and post hoc analyses focuses on identifying the ideal decompensated HF patient population most likely to benefit from AVP receptor antagonism in terms of acute decongestion and short-term outcomes and aids in identifying knowledge gaps to be addressed in future prospective clinical trials.

ROLE OF AVP IN HYPONATREMIA AND HF

AVP, also known as antidiuretic hormone (ADH), is a neuropeptide that has the primary physiologic function of regulating the body's water and sodium balance and volume homeostasis. It is synthesized in the hypothalamus and stored in the posterior pituitary. Under normal physiologic conditions, AVP is secreted in response to increased plasma osmolality and significantly reduced arterial pressure or blood volume.[4,29] In the circulation, AVP exerts effects at 3 different receptors (V1a, V1b, and V2) located at different sites and cells of the body.

Binding of AVP to V1a and V2 receptor subtypes has been theorized to contribute to the natural history of HF because of regulation of vascular tone, cardiovascular (CV) contractility, and body fluid status.[4–6,29,30] Binding of AVP at V1a-receptors in the vascular smooth muscle cells and cardiomyocytes induces vasoconstriction and cardiac contractility, respectively. Binding of AVP at V2-receptors in the renal collecting duct induces reabsorption of free water back into circulation via increased expression and insertion of aquaporin (AQP-2) channels to restore volume homeostasis and decrease plasma osmolality. If unregulated, increased AVP binding at V2-receptors could lead to increased water retention, while sodium continues to be excreted in the urine, resulting in dilutional hyponatremia.

Based on registry data and clinical trial experience, hyponatremia occurs in 10% to 27% of patients hospitalized with HF; on average, baseline serum sodium (Na) has been low (137-138 mEq/L) in patients hospitalized for HF.[2,3,20,31,32] Among patients admitted for acute decompensated heart failure (ADHF), those with serum sodium less than 135 to 137 mEq/L at admission have shown significantly reduced survival than those with normonatremia at admission.[1,2,31,32] In the Outcomes of a Prospective Trial of Intravenous Milrinone for Exacerbations of Chronic Heart Failure (OPTIME-CHF) study, 27% of patients had serum Na less than 137 mEq/L at baseline; baseline serum sodium was shown to be an independent predictor of 60-day outcomes in this population with left ventricular (LV) systolic dysfunction.[2] Severe hyponatremia was associated with a high event rate of death or rehospitalization (41%) at 60 days. Analysis of the Organized Program to Initiate Lifesaving Treatment in Hospitalized Patients with Heart Failure (OPTIMIZE-HF) registry showed that hyponatremia

(Na <135 mEq/L) was associated with significantly higher rates of in-hospital mortality and longer hospital length of stays (LOS), regardless of LV dysfunction.[1] Interestingly, rehospitalization rates at 60 to 90 days were equally high regardless of serum sodium at admission in OPTIMIZE-HF, although correction of serum sodium at discharge was not analyzed and correlated to rates of rehospitalization.

In HF, neurohormonal imbalance with elevated levels of norepinephrine, angiotensin-II, aldosterone, endothelin, and AVP have all been shown to induce vasoconstriction, tachycardia, and fluid retention.[4,33] Given the role of AVP in neurohormonal activation and water retention, plasma AVP concentration has been shown to be significantly and chronically elevated in patients with HF, particularly in those with hyponatremia and decompensated HF.[30] Baseline evaluation of the Studies of Left Ventricular Dysfunction (SOLVD) database showed an incremental increase in plasma AVP concentrations from healthy individuals to asymptomatic patients and symptomatic patients with HF due to LV dysfunction.[33] Due to AVP's role in the modulation of several processes implicated in the pathogenesis of HF, several large, randomized clinical trials have studied AVP receptor antagonists in HF and have demonstrated promising short-term efficacy and long-term safety profile with their use. However, no prospective trial has targeted patients with HF and hyponatremia until recently.

DEVELOPMENT OF AVP RECEPTOR ANTAGONISTS ("VAPTANS")

Over the past decade, the development of vaptans has advanced the management of dilutional hyponatremia from conventional methods that were marginally effective and poorly tolerated. Compared with conventional treatments such as strict fluid restriction (<800 mL/d), hypertonic saline, and loop diuresis, vaptans have demonstrated significant efficacy in correction of serum sodium in patients with hypervolemic and euvolemic hyponatremia without inducing electrolyte imbalance or worsening renal function.[7] Although dietary sodium restriction and diuretic therapy remain the mainstays of therapy for all diseases associated with edema formation, AVP antagonism is a viable therapy for hypervolemic hyponatremia because excess AVP secretion appears to be the most important pathophysiological factor involved in these conditions.[29] Both tolvaptan and conivaptan exert their main pharmacologic effects at the V2-receptors in the renal collecting duct.

Studies have shown that tolvaptan, a selective V2-receptor antagonist, and conivaptan, a dual V1a/V2-receptor antagonist, both substantially increase aquaresis and plasma osmolality.[7–9] Both agents are indicated for the treatment of clinically significant hypervolemic and euvolemic hyponatremia, including patients with HF and syndrome of inappropriate antidiuretic hormone (SIADH) to correct serum sodium concentrations.[10,11] Underlying conditions, such as HF, cirrhosis, and renal failure, are commonly associated with hypervolemic hyponatremia, whereas SIADH is commonly associated with euvolemic hyponatremia.[29] Despite the approval of vaptans for treating hyponatremia, long-term survival benefit due to correction of hyponatremia remains unknown. Although neither agent is indicated for the treatment of congestive or decompensated HF, both have demonstrated increased net fluid loss without causing electrolyte imbalance in patients with HF, regardless of serum sodium concentrations at baseline.[13,14,16–19] In addition to favorable tolerability and safety profiles, several post hoc analyses of the trials with tolvaptan in HF have suggested some interesting hypotheses regarding the therapeutic niche of tolvaptan to provide favorable clinical outcomes in target patients.

ADHF

With better appreciation of the role of neurohormonal activation in HF, drugs inhibiting the renin-angiotensin-aldosterone system and sympathetic nervous system have become the standard of care based on safety, efficacy, and improvements in outcomes from pivotal landmark clinical trials. Unfortunately, these therapeutic agents are not enough to reduce mortality and morbidity associated with ADHF; patients hospitalized for HF are at especially high risk for death and rehospitalization in the early period after discharge.[34,35]

Characterization of patients hospitalized for ADHF indicates that most patients with HF are admitted with evidence of volume overload, including signs and symptoms of dyspnea at rest or on minimal exertion, weight gain, orthopnea, paroxysmal nocturnal dyspnea, jugular venous distension (JVD), rales, and peripheral edema.[31,36] Goals of therapy are thus to improve signs and symptoms of congestion, identify precipitating factors and cause of ADHF, minimize adverse effects of therapy, and optimize chronic therapy to prevent neurohormonal imbalance and rehospitalization. Conventional strategies, such as fluid and sodium restriction, have been shown to be difficult to manage and maintain in patients. Other therapeutic strategies for ADHF include loop diuresis, inotropes, vasodilators and natriuretic peptide, and ultrafiltration (UF) to mechanically remove sodium and water. However, effective strategies are often limited by short-term and long-term complications. Chronic renal insufficiency has been shown to be present in 30% of patients with HF, and 20% of these patients have serum creatinine (SCr) greater than 2.0 mg/dL at hospital admission.[37] Patients hospitalized for ADHF with severe dyspnea, altered mental status, decreased systolic blood pressure (SBP), and worsening renal function are generally poor candidates for loop diuretic therapy and are left with limited treatment options. UF may be an option for patients with diuretic resistance and renal impairment, but in a prospective, randomized, placebo-controlled trial of 200 patients with ADHF due to overload, UF did not improve dyspnea relief at 48 hours.[38] Use of nesiritide in the ADHF population was shown to improve dyspnea relief, but controversy and uncertainty remain regarding nesiritide's effect on 30-day outcomes.[39,40]

Because of the lack of effective strategies to consistently demonstrate improvements in congestive symptoms and clinical outcomes, therapeutic agents for ADHF have not changed significantly over the past decades. In patients hospitalized for ADHF with evidence of significant volume overload, intravenous (IV) loop diuretics remain first-line therapy, and urine output and signs and symptoms of congestion should be serially assessed to guide adjustment of diuretic dose.[21] However, loop diuretics induce isotonic urine output and may worsen hyponatremia and renal function.[29,41] Risk stratification for in-hospital mortality from the Acute Decompensated Heart Failure National Registry (ADHERE) showed that the strongest predictors on admission for increased mortality were high levels of blood urea nitrogen (BUN $\geq$43 mg/dL), SBP less than 115 mm Hg, and SCr greater than or equal to 2.75 mg/dL.[37] Data from the OPTIMIZE-HF registry confirmed lower SBP, elevated SCr, and BUN, and admission and discharge serum sodium as predictors of after discharge mortality.[36] Given that loop diuretic therapy has been associated with increased risk of hypotension, electrolyte abnormalities, and even mortality, the unmet need for the development of novel agents for successful treatment of ADHF is substantial.[42,43]

Review of Clinical Evidence for Vaptans Approved in the United States

Two vaptans, conivaptan and tolvaptan, have been extensively studied and have shown efficacy in patients with hyponatremia. Tolvaptan has also been well studied in patients hospitalized with acute HF and in outpatients with chronic HF.[19,20,44]

CONIVAPTAN

Conivaptan, a vasopressin antagonist that reversibly binds to both V1a and V2 receptors with a 10:1 binding affinity, was approved by the FDA for the IV treatment of euvolemic hyponatremia in 2005 and hypervolemic hyponatremia in 2007.[10] In a randomized, double-blind, placebo-controlled, phase III study of 84 hospitalized patients with euvolemic (N = 56) or hypervolemic (N = 28), hyponatremia from a variety of underlying causes and disease conditions, including CHF, IV administration of conivaptan 40 mg/d for 4 days increased aquaresis and serum sodium levels.[9] Oral conivaptan (40 or 80 mg/d in 2 divided doses) has also demonstrated significant dose-dependent improvements in serum sodium compared with placebo in patients with euvolemic and hypervolemic hyponatremia; however, the oral formulation (absolute bioavailability of 44%) has not been approved in the United States.[8]

In patients with CHF, conivaptan has shown favorable hemodynamic impact but has not demonstrated efficacy for treating signs and symptoms of HF. In a multicenter, randomized, double-blind, placebo-controlled clinical trial, 142 patients with New York Heart Association (NYHA) class III/IV HF due to LV systolic dysfunction were randomized to receive a single IV dose of placebo or conivaptan (10, 20, or 40 mg).[12] Conivaptan 20 and 40 mg were shown to significantly reduce pulmonary capillary wedge pressure (PCWP) and right atrial pressure compared with placebo ($P<.05$). Other hemodynamic parameters, such as cardiac index, systemic vascular resistance (SVR), blood pressure (BP), and heart rate (HR), did not differ significantly between treatment groups. In a multicenter, double-blind, placebo-controlled, dose-ranging pilot study, 170 patients hospitalized for worsening CHF were randomized to 2 successive 24-hour infusions of placebo or conivaptan (40, 80, or 120 mg/d) in addition to standard therapy.[13] Conivaptan was effective in increasing urine output compared with standard of care diuretic therapy up to 72 hours; there was a trend toward a greater body weight reduction with each dosage group compared with placebo, although not statistically significantly. However, conivaptan did not improve dyspnea or clinical signs and symptoms of congestion compared with placebo at 48 hours, which was the primary endpoint of the study. The mean serum sodium was significantly increased at each time point in each of the conivaptan groups compared with placebo, and this serum sodium increase was also dose-proportional.

TOLVAPTAN

Tolvaptan is an oral selective AVP V2-receptor antagonist that has been approved by the FDA for the treatment of euvolemic or hypervolemic hyponatremia (serum Na <135 mEq/L) based on statistically significant improvements in serum sodium concentrations from baseline to day 4 and day 30 in the Study of Ascending Levels of Tolvaptan in Hyponatremia 1 and 2 (SALT-1 and SALT-2) trials.[7] In fact, serum sodium concentrations were significantly higher in the tolvaptan group than in the placebo group within 8 hours after the initial dose. This difference was seen throughout the treatment period of 30 days, but not at 1 week after discontinuation of study drug, indicating that the aquaretic effect of tolvaptan may be required to maintain a normal sodium concentration in patients with chronic hyponatremia. In the SALT trials, 31% of patients had chronic HF, 27% had cirrhosis, and 42% of patients had SIADH or other conditions causing hyponatremia at baseline. In terms of secondary measures that were pertinent to HF, net fluid loss and body weight reduction were statistically significantly greater with tolvaptan compared to placebo on day 1. Since randomization was stratified according to severity of hyponatremia and presence of underlying HF, data or post hoc analysis of this group of nearly 140 patients with chronic HF and hyponatremia might have provided useful observations about the effect of tolvaptan or sodium correction on the clinical course in this population over the 30-day study period. However, outcome measures were not studied in the SALT trials.

TOLVAPTAN IN HF

Tolvaptan has been studied in patients with stable HF as well as decompensated HF for over ten years. A comparison of these major trials is described in this section and summarized in **Table 1**. In a proof of concept (PoC) outpatient study in 254 patients (28% of whom had serum Na ≤136 mEq/L at baseline) with NYHA I–III HF, regardless of LVEF, treatment with tolvaptan (30, 45, or 60 mg once daily) showed a statistically significant greater body weight reduction than placebo on day 1 (P<.001), which was maintained throughout the study with no additional weight reduction observed.[16] A greater mean net fluid loss was also observed with tolvaptan than placebo on day 1 (P<.05 at each dose); and this was not dose-dependent. Based on pharmacokinetic

(PK) and pharmacodynamic (PD) studies of tolvaptan in healthy volunteers, the aquaretic effect of tolvaptan was shown not to be dose-proportional due to a saturation of the aquaretic response.[45,46]

In a dose-ranging phase II feasibility study, the Acute and Chronic Therapeutic Impact of a Vasopressin Antagonist in Congestive Heart Failure (ACTIV in CHF), the effects of tolvaptan on short-term clinical course and 60-day outcomes in 319 hospitalized patients with reduced LVEF and persistent congestion were investigated.[17] Again, tolvaptan was shown to reduce body weight at 24 hours (one of the co-primary endpoints) without worsening renal function or affecting serum potassium and vital signs; and this effect was independent of the dose. Unlike the outpatient study aforementioned, ACTIV in CHF only enrolled decompensated HF patients with LVEF less than or equal to 40%.

Although no adjustments in α significance level were made for the co-primary endpoint analysis and multiple comparisons (each dosing group vs placebo), tolvaptan clearly demonstrated increased net fluid loss and reduced body weight more effectively than standard therapy alone. However, the study did not show a difference in rate of worsening HF at 60 days between patients treated with tolvaptan versus placebo (26.7% vs 27.5%). Death by 60 days was 5.4% in the 3 tolvaptan groups combined and 8.7% in placebo (P = .18). The authors also reported from a prespecified post hoc analysis that mortality might be reduced in high-risk patients (with elevated BUN levels and severe systemic congestion) treated with tolvaptan.[13] However, the analysis was not reported in detail and the study was not powered to confidently report this observation.

Along with renal insufficiency and severe systemic congestion, baseline hyponatremia has also been established as a prognostic marker for worse outcomes in patients hospitalized for worsening HF in clinical trials.[2,3] Of the patients with baseline serum sodium data from ACTIV in CHF, 22% (69/301) had hyponatremia (Na ≤135 mEq/L) at admission and were included in a post hoc analysis.[25] The data confirmed baseline hyponatremia as an independent predictor of 60-day mortality, after adjustment for covariates. Patients randomized to tolvaptan (n = 52) experienced early and sustained improvements in serum sodium concentrations that were not evident in the placebo group (n = 16). The 60-day mortality among patients with improved serum sodium was 11.1% (5/45) compared with 21.7% (5/23) in hyponatremic patients whose serum sodium did not improve. Pooled analysis of treatment with multiple doses of tolvaptan was associated with

Table 1
Comparison of key similarities and differences in clinical trials and post hoc analyses with tolvaptan in HF

Clinical Trial	Study Design	Target Population	Sample Size	Study Endpoints	Study Results
SALT 1,2 (phase III)	Multicenter, placebo-controlled, double-blind, dose-escalating (15–60 mg/d) for 30 d	Euvolemic or hypervolemic hyponatremia (Na <135 mEq/L) 31% of patients had chronic HF	N = 448; SBP ≥90; SCr ≤3.5	1° endpoints: change in serum sodium from baseline to day 4 and from baseline to day 30. Pertinent 2° measures (to HF): net fluid loss and change in body weight (BW) on day 1	Increased serum sodium at days 4 and 30; faster correction of serum sodium during hospitalization. No changes in renal function and serum electrolyte concentrations
Gheorghiade et al,[16] 2003 (POC study)	Placebo-controlled, double-blind, multidose (30, 45, 60 mg/d) for 25 d	Chronic HF NYHA I–III regardless of LVEF; baseline oral furosemide therapy 40–240 mg/d at least 7 d before enrollment	N = 254; SCr ≤3.0	1° endpoints: change in BW from baseline to day 14. 2° measures: edema, urine sodium excretion, urine osmolality, and net fluid loss	More BW reduction at 24 h at all dose levels and was sustained throughout the study with no additional benefit. More net fluid loss at 24 h at all dose levels. No changes in vital signs, renal function, or serum potassium
ACTIV in CHF (phase II feasibility)	Placebo-controlled, double-blind, multidose (30, 60, 90 mg/d) for up to 60 d	ADHF and LVEF ≤40%; randomized within 96 h	N = 319; SBP ≥110; SCr ≤3.0	1° endpoints: change in BW at 24 h and evidence of worsening HF at 60 d. 2° measures: changes in dyspnea, JVD, rales, edema, and discharge BW from baseline. urine output (UO), serum electrolyte levels, use of diuretics, index hospital LOS	More reduction in BW at 24 h. No difference in 60-d outcomes in the overall population
High-risk patients post hoc analysis	Analysis not reported in detail	Elevated BUN and severe systemic congestion			60-d outcomes benefit in high-risk group with tolvaptan
Hyponatremia post hoc analysis		21% (68/319) with hyponatremia (Na ≤ 136) vs normonatremia			60-d mortality benefit in patients with hyponatremia who received tolvaptan

Trial/Reference	Design	Population	N	Endpoints/Measures	Results
Udelson et al,[18] 2007	Multicenter, randomized, double-blind, placebo-controlled study with administration of tolvaptan (30 mg/d) or placebo for up to 1 y	NYHA II-III and LVEF ≤40%	N = 240, SBP ≥90, SCr ≤3.0	1° endpoints: change left ventricular end-diastolic volume (LVEDV) after 1 y of therapy, and repeated again ~1 wk after withdrawal of study drug. 2° measures: LVESV, LVEF, vital signs, renal function, serum Na and K, global status and respiratory symptoms. Deaths and HF-hospitalizations	Small, nonsignificant reduction in LVEDV between treatment groups after 1 y. Significant favorable effect of tolvaptan on the composite of mortality or HF-hospitalizations. No differences in serum electrolytes or renal function; no differences in symptoms
ECLIPSE	Multicenter, randomized, placebo-controlled, double-blind study with single oral dose of tolvaptan (15, 30, or 60 mg) or placebo	NYHA III-IV and LVEF <40%	N = 181, SBP ≥90, SCr ≤3.0	1° measures: acute hemodynamic parameters: PCWP, right atrial pressure (RAP), pulmonary arterial pressure, vitals (BP, HR), PVR, SVR, cardiac index. 2° measures: UO, renal function, urine osmolality, serum Na, K	Tolvaptan at all doses significantly reduced PCWP. Only 15- or 30-mg doses significantly reduced RAP. No changes in cardiac index, SVR, PVR, or vital signs were observed. Tolvaptan significantly increased UO by 3 h in a dose-dependent manner without affecting renal function, serum electrolytes
EVEREST (phase III)	Multicenter, randomized, placebo-controlled, double-blind trial to study the effect of tolvaptan (30 mg/d) in 2 clinical-course trials embedded in an outcomes trial	ADHF and LVEF ≤40%; randomized within 48 h	N = 4133, SBP ≥90, SCr ≤3.5	1° endpoints: composite of changes in global clinical status (VAS) and BW at day 7 or discharge; time to all-cause mortality and CV-mortality or HF-hospitalization. 2° measures: VAS day 1, signs and symptoms of congestion on day 7 or discharge	Met composite primary endpoint largely driven by increased BW loss with tolvaptan; significant dyspnea relief and BW lost at day 1 with tolvaptan. No outcomes benefit with tolvaptan. No changes in vital signs, renal function, or serum potassium
Hyponatremia post hoc analysis		Hyponatremia (Na < 135), and subset of marked hyponatremia (Na < 130)	N = 475 with Na < 135, N = 92 with Na < 130		Patients with Na <130 had favorable outcomes of reduced CV-mortality/morbidity. No difference in outcomes in overall hyponatremia (Na <135) patients

a reduction in 60-day mortality compared with placebo. Furthermore, 60-day mortality was statistically significantly lower in hyponatremic patients who received tolvaptan than those who received placebo.

TOLVAPTAN—PHASE III EVEREST PROGRAM AND ANALYSES

The Efficacy of Vasopressin Antagonism in Heart Failure Outcome Study with Tolvaptan (EVEREST) Program was designed to be 2 identical short-term studies embedded in one large outcomes trial with 2 co-primary outcomes endpoints of all-cause mortality and CV-related mortality or HF-related hospitalizations.[19,20] It was also one of the first and largest trials designed to explore appropriate clinical endpoints and assess outcomes benefit in the decompensated HF patient population; and lessons have been derived from its design, execution, and subgroup analyses.

The EVEREST Program was a prospective, international, randomized, double-blind, placebo-controlled clinical trial that also targeted patients with LVEF less than or equal to 40%, same as in ACTIV in CHF, who were hospitalized for worsening HF and had signs and symptoms of volume overload. Four thousand one hundred thirty-three eligible patients were randomized within 48 hours of presentation to either placebo or tolvaptan (30 mg/d) in addition to standard IV loop diuretic therapy and treated up to 7 days. Co-primary endpoints and secondary measures are outlined in **Table 1**. Rank sum analysis of the composite primary endpoint showed a significantly greater improvement with tolvaptan than placebo in both trials ($P<.001$), but this benefit was driven primarily by changes in body weight. In terms of immediate clinical benefits on inpatient day 1, greater improvements were observed in the tolvaptan groups for both body weight reductions ($P<.001$) and dyspnea relief ($P<.0001$) from baseline. In the trial design, timing of the day 1 study visit could be performed at any time on the calendar day after the first dose of study drug. Thus, the timing of patient-reported dyspnea in relation to the first dose of study medication varied by patient and since patients were randomized up to 48 hours post-admission, time points for the data were largely variable, from several hours to 72 hours post-initial presentation of worsening HF. Given the heterogenous baseline characteristics of the patient population in EVEREST, prespecified subgroups were analyzed to help identify better responders to tolvaptan treatment as well as explore more appropriate clinical endpoints for tolvaptan's optimal therapeutic window to account

for its relatively quick onset of action and aquaretic threshold.

Although dyspnea is the most common chief complaint in patients hospitalized for ADHF, the assessment of changes in this symptom has not been well studied. Post hoc analysis from EVEREST has shown that tolvaptan's effects on patient-reported dyspnea relief were greatest within 12 hours after first dose (lasting until 20 hours) when added to standard therapy with IV loop diuretics; and modest improvements were maintained up to 60 hours after admission.[23] This is somewhat related to tolvaptan's PD effect for decongestion. In healthy subjects, tolvaptan has shown an increased aquaretic effect within two to four hours post-dose; but urine output was similar across a range of doses within 12 hours post-dose.[45,46] Patient-reported dyspnea was also shown to be associated with physician-assessed measurements of congestion (orthopnea, JVD, edema, and body weight). Post hoc analysis on these measures demonstrated a greater likelihood of clinical improvement among tolvaptan-treated patients as early as inpatient day 1 and lasting through day 3 for orthopnea and day 7 for JVD.[24]

In EVEREST, patients were not stratified based on baseline serum sodium, but the short-term clinical course of patients with hyponatremia (Na <135mEq/L) at baseline and the effects of tolvaptan on outcomes have been reported in a recent post hoc analysis.[26] Among the 475 patients with hyponatremia at baseline, there was no effect of tolvaptan on all-cause mortality or CV-related outcomes compared with placebo. In a smaller subset of 92 patients with marked hyponatremia (Na <130 mEq/L), treatment with tolvaptan (n = 38) was associated with reduced CV-related death or hospitalization when compared with placebo (n = 54) (hazard ratio [HR] 0.60 [95% confidence interval (CI): 0.37-0.98] $P = .04$). This improvement was not seen with similar statistical significance in CV-death or HF-hospitalization (HR 0.69 [95% CI: 0.42-1.12] $P = .21$), or all-cause mortality (HR 0.76 [95% CI: 0.44-1.29] $P = .34$). Interestingly, in the placebo group, patients with hyponatremia at baseline had less dyspnea relief compared with the normonatremia cohort on day 1 (59.2% vs 69.2%; $P<.01$), despite higher diuretic dosing, which reached significant difference beginning inpatient day 3 ($P<.05$). The authors did not adjust the analysis for covariates due to the small sample size; the observation needs validation in prospective studies to determine if serum sodium correction during hospitalization actually improves outcomes as opposed to solely being a marker for worse outcomes in patients with HF and hyponatremia.

To date, only post hoc analyses have evaluated the effects of sodium correction in HF patients with symptomatic volume overload and outcomes. These results have suggested that tolvaptan may be a useful and valuable adjunct therapy for decongestion in patients with ADHF, particularly in those with hyponatremia and/or chronic renal insufficiency. However, inconsistent endpoints and target patient populations have complicated clinical trial data, and a well-defined, optimal therapeutic window for the use of tolvaptan in HF remains to be identified.

TOLVAPTAN—FAVORABLE SAFETY, TOLERABILITY, AND HEMODYNAMIC PROFILES

One concern with the use of tolvaptan was the displacement of AVP from V2-receptors to increased stimulation of the V1a receptor, resulting in vasoconstriction in the peripheral and coronary circulations. In a multicenter study that evaluated the hemodynamic effects of long-term administration of tolvaptan or placebo in 240 patients with reduced LVEF, while AVP levels were higher in patients treated with tolvaptan than with placebo, the data showed no significant changes in LV volumes with one year of tolvaptan therapy, ruling out the possibility of unopposed V1a-receptor stimulation during chronic selective V2-receptor antagonism.[18] Interestingly, while there was only a trend towards symptom improvement with tolvaptan therapy, the data have suggested a statistically significant favorable association of tolvaptan on the composite of mortality or HF-related hospitalizations. However, the effect on natural history outcomes was not prespecified, and clinical events were not adjudicated to a specific outcomes committee. There was no difference in the number of patients withdrawn from the trial due to AEs or serious AEs. The most commonly reported side effects with tolvaptan were increased urinary frequency, thirst, and dry mouth, which were consistent with previously reported common AEs from EVEREST and a year long, open-label extension of the SALT trials.[22]

The ECLIPSE (EffeCt of toLvaptan on hemodynamIc Parameters in Subjects with hEart failure) study further provided mechanistic support for the symptomatic improvements noted with tolvaptan in patients with decompensated HF and reduced LVEF.[15] A single dose of tolvaptan resulted in modest but favorable changes in filling pressures and pulmonary artery pressures that were not dose-dependent. These changes occurred with no significant effects on other hemodynamic parameters, serum electrolyte levels, or renal function. Udelson and colleagues[12,15] have suggested that considering the similar results from the hemodynamic studies of tolvaptan and conivaptan, the predominant clinical effects of vaptans are mediated by V2-receptor antagonism, even for the dual-receptor antagonist conivaptan. The lack of adverse effect on remodeling observed with chronic oral tolvaptan therapy for up to 1 year also suggests that a chronic V1a-receptor effect during V2-receptor antagonism by tolvaptan would not be clinically concerning in patients with HF.[15]

TARGETED CLINICAL TRIAL DESIGN AND FUTURE STUDIES OF TOLVAPTAN IN HF

Therapeutic management of ADHF in patients with hyponatremia, renal insufficiency, and refractory diuresis is challenging and associated with unfavorable clinical outcomes. Clinical evidence has suggested an important role and therapeutic potential for the use of tolvaptan in this high-risk ADHF patient population. Furthermore, economic cost-offset analyses of results from the SALT trials and EVEREST have suggested that the observed reductions in LOS were associated with substantial estimated mean hospital cost reductions in patients with HF.[47,48] Interest remains high in identifying the ideal decompensated HF patient population that may benefit most from tolvaptan in terms of symptom relief, decongestion, and clinical outcomes.

A review and comparison of prior clinical trials with tolvaptan in HF (see **Table 1**) have suggested several modifications and improvements in study designs for prospective trials that target decompensated HF patients with reduced serum sodium. Eligibility criteria for past clinical trials in decompensated HF typically did not include an elevated b-type natriuretic peptide (BNP) or N-terminal of the prohormone BNP (NT-proBNP) requirement. Natriuretic peptide is a strong prognostic factor for patients hospitalized for worsening HF, and inclusion of a BNP/NT-proBNP requirement would provide better documentation of volume overload to solidify evidence of congestion.[21,49] Given the role of dyspnea relief in regulatory approval due to its prevalence as a chief complaint in patients seeking medical care for worsening HF, it has become a consistent target in acute HF clinical trials. However, the scale of measurement has not been well defined. Nesiritide has demonstrated statistically significant improvement in dyspnea, whereas serelaxin improved dyspnea by the VAS but not by the trial's other primary endpoint by the Likert scale.[39,50] The primary dyspnea endpoint in EVEREST was

Table 2
Comparison of ongoing clinical trials of tolvaptan in decompensated HF with EVEREST

	TACTICS-HF (Target N = 250)	SECRET-CHF (Target N = 250)	EVEREST (Actual N = 4133)
Randomization and therapy	Randomized within 24 h of presentation. Treatment up to 3 d in-hospital	Randomized within 36 h of presentation. Treatment up to 7 d in-hospital	Randomized within 48 h of presentation; treated up to 7 d in-hospital
Eligibility (inclusion/exclusion criteria)	History of CHF, regardless of LVEF. Decompensated HF as determined by dyspnea at rest/minimum exertion or NT-proBNP >2000 pg/mL AND ≥1 of the following: • Orthopnea • Elevated JVD • Peripheral edema • Congestion on CXR • Pulmonary rales SBP ≥90 SCr ≤3.5 and not on dialysis Na ≤140 mEq/L Prior treatment with loop diuretic therapy for at least 40 mg furosemide daily for at least 30 d	History of CHF, regardless of LVEF NYHA III–IV (moderate to severe dyspnea) and volume overload as based on ≥2 of the following: • Elevated JVD • Pitting edema • Ascites • Congestion on CXR • Pulmonary rales No NT-proBNP criteria SBP ≥90 SCr ≤3.5 and not on dialysis AND ≥1 of the following: • Renal insufficiency (estimated glomerular filtration rate <60 mL/min/1.73 m²) • Hyponatremia (Na ≤134) • Loop diuretic resistance as evidenced by reduced UO following IV furosemide ≥40 mg based on defined cumulative UO over time	History of CHF and LVEF ≤40%. Congestion based on signs and symptoms of volume overload based on ≥2 of the following: • Dyspnea at rest/minimum exertion • Elevated JVD • Pitting edema No NT-proBNP criteria SBP ≥90 SCr ≤3.5 and not on dialysis No serum Na requirement K ≤5.5 mEq/L Hemoglobin <9 g/dL
1° Endpoints	Coprimary endpoints of % of patients with at least moderate improvement in dyspnea at both 8 and 24 h (Likert scale); without need for rescue therapy at 24 h	Dyspnea improvement at 8 and 16 h by Likert scale	Composite of changes in global clinical status (VAS) and BW at day 7 or discharge; all-cause mortality and CV-related hospitalizations and/or mortality
2° Measures	Change in renal function; BW and net fluid loss at day 7 or discharge; hospital LOS; % of patients with persistent/worsen HF; 30-day outcomes (death/ED/rehospitalization)	Change in renal function at day 7 or discharge; daily diuretic use; hospital LOS; change in cognition at 48 h or discharge; 30-day outcomes (death/ED/rehospitalization)	Changes in dyspnea (day 1), BW (days 1 and 7 or discharge), physician-assessed signs and symptoms (day 7 or discharge), and patient-assessed VAS (day 7 or discharge)

on day 7 instead of day 1, when tolvaptan has consistently demonstrated the most effect in body weight reduction and net fluid loss on day 1. Secondary endpoint showed tolvaptan significantly reduced dyspnea on day 1 compared with placebo, and analysis has suggested that the maximal dyspnea relief with tolvaptan occurs at 12 hours after the first dose, lasting until 20 hours, followed by a modest improvement up to 60 hours after first dose.[23] Correlations analysis showed that physician-assessed measurements of congestion, such as orthopnea, JVD, edema, and body weight, were associated with patient-assessed dyspnea. There was a linear association between reductions in body weight and improvements in dyspnea, a finding to be confirmed in prospective trials.[23,24] Also, administration of tolvaptan was widely varied and generally given late after presentation in past clinical trials because of a wide randomization window. Slightly earlier administration may help standardize variability in dyspnea assessments from actual presentation to the hospital for ADHF.

Because patients with HF are at significantly high risk for mortality and rehospitalization in the early period after index hospital discharge, a 30-day to 60-day endpoint HF-related mortality and morbidity may be an appropriate measure of short-term clinical outcomes. Analysis of the OPTIMIZE-HF registry showed high event rates of 8.6% mortality and 29.6% rehospitalization within 60 to 90 days after discharge; composite endpoint of mortality and/or rehospitalization was 36.2%.[31,35] Sixty-day mortality was shown to be 8.9% to 10.3% in OPTIME-CHF.[2,32] Furthermore, none of the available or investigative therapeutic strategies have been able to improve outcomes in terms of reduction in rehospitalizations, unscheduled clinic or ED visits, or mortality.

Two ongoing investigator-initiated, prospective, multicenter, randomized, double-blind, placebo-controlled feasibility studies are ongoing to evaluate the effects of tolvaptan as adjunct therapy to standard of care IV loop diuretics in symptomatic HF patients with hyponatremia, and chronic renal insufficiency whose volume status may be difficult to manage with oral loop diuretics.[27,28] Each study is targeted to enroll 250 patients admitted with ADHF and evidence of volume overload. Unlike ACTIV in CHF and EVEREST that only enrolled patients with reduced LVEF, these 2 ongoing trials are enrolling patients with ADHF, regardless of LVEF. A comparison of these studies is outlined in **Table 2**.

The Targeting Acute Congestion with Tolvaptan In CongeStive Heart Failure (TACTICS-HF) study is an investigator-initiated clinical trial designed to compare the effects of oral tolvaptan versus placebo as an adjunct therapy to fixed-dose IV furosemide on dyspnea relief, renal function, and changes in clinical status in patients hospitalized with ADHF. The study is enrolling patients hospitalized for ADHF with signs and symptoms of volume overload and NT-proBNP greater than 2000 pg/mL.[27] Patients are randomized within 24 hours of presentation to placebo or tolvaptan 30 mg/d in addition to IV loop diuretics and treated up to 3 days in-hospital. The primary endpoint is the proportion of patients with at least moderate improvement in dyspnea at both 8 and 24 hours, and without need for rescue therapy for worsening HF at 24 hours. Secondary measures of the study include change in renal function, body weight and net fluid loss, hospital LOS, percentage of patients with persistent or worsening HF, and 30-day clinical outcomes.

The Study to Evaluate Challenging REsponders to Therapy in Congestive Heart Failure Trial (SECRET of CHF) is designed to evaluate the short-term efficacy and safety of tolvaptan in subjects hospitalized for worsening HF who have volume overload and either concurrent hyponatremia (Na <135 mEq/L), renal insufficiency (estimated glomerular filtration rate (eGFR) <60 mL/min/1.73 m^2), or insufficient response to initial IV diuretic therapy.[28] Patients are randomized within 36 hours of presentation to placebo or tolvaptan 30 mg/d in addition to IV loop diuretics and treated up to 7 days in-hospital. The primary endpoint is a composite of patient-reported dyspnea improvement (Likert scale) at 8 and 16 hours after first dose. Secondary measures of the study include change in renal function at day 7 or discharge, change in cognitive function at 48 hours or discharge, diuretic use, hospital LOS, and 30-day clinical outcomes. This study will likely allow for subgroup analysis to compare patients with HF and one or more of these predictors of worse outcomes. The goals of this clinical trial are primarily to demonstrate that tolvaptan as an adjunct therapy for standard of care treatment of ADHF will result in better and more rapid volume homeostasis, and thus more rapid relief of symptoms. Secondary goals are to reduce the likelihood of worsening renal function by decreasing the need for escalation of loop diuretic therapy to achieve decongestion and net fluid loss.

SUMMARY

Although progress has been made to reduce mortality associated with HF, rates of HF-related hospitalizations (associated with cardiac and/or renal injury) continue to increase, approaching 30%

within 30 to 60 days after discharge.[49] Hyponatremia is a known complication in HF; patients with reduced serum sodium concentrations, lower SBP, severe congestion, and renal insufficiency at admission are difficult to manage with current standard of care with IV loop diuresis, contributing to their poor prognoses.

Tolvaptan, an orally active selective AVP V2-receptor antagonist that increases aquaresis, has been approved for the treatment of euvolemic or hypervolemic hyponatremia in patients, including those with underlying disease of HF.[11] Despite not improving outcomes in patients with decompensated HF, tolvaptan remains a potential option in managing decongestion without adversely affecting renal function, serum electrolyte concentrations, and hemodynamics. Clinical trials in patients with decompensated HF have demonstrated tolvaptan's increased efficacy for greater body weight reduction and net fluid loss at 24 hours in addition to standard loop diuretic therapy.[17–20]

TACTICS-HF and SECRET in CHF are 2 ongoing prospective trials that target more defined patient populations with decompensated HF and aim to test the hypotheses generated from analyses described in this article. The results from these trials will help define the role of tolvaptan in HF and its optimal use in challenging patients with HF, hyponatremia, renal insufficiency, and/or loop diuretic resistance, with, it is hoped, a decrease in hospital admissions at 30 days in this high-risk patient population. It is conceivable that with multiple doses or recurrent use of tolvaptan, volume homeostasis may be maintained at lower doses of loop diuretic therapy in patients, lowering the risk of worsening renal function.

REFERENCES

1. Gheorghiade M, Abraham WT, Albert NM, et al. Relationship between admission serum sodium concentration and clinical outcomes in patients hospitalized for heart failure: an analysis from the OPTIMIZE-HF registry. Eur Heart J 2007;28(8):980–8.
2. Klein L, O'Connor CM, Leimberger JD, et al. Lower serum sodium is associated with increased short-term mortality in hospitalized patients with worsening heart failure: results from the Outcomes of a Prospective Trial of Intravenous Milrinone for Exacerbations of Chronic Heart Failure (OPTIME-CHF) study. Circulation 2005;111(19):2454–60.
3. Gheorghiade M, Hellkamp A, Pina IL, et al. Characterization and prognostic value of persistent hyponatremia in patients with severe heart failure in the ESCAPE trial. Arch Intern Med 2007;167(18):1998–2005.
4. Lee CR, Watkins ML, Patterson JH, et al. Vasopressin: a new target for the treatment of heart failure. Am Heart J 2003;146:9–18.
5. Finley JJ IV, Konstam MA, Udelson JE. Arginine vasopressin antagonists for the treatment of heart failure and hyponatremia. Circulation 2008;118:410–21.
6. Oghlakian G, Klapholz M. Vasopressin and vasopressin receptor antagonists in heart failure. Cardiol Rev 2009;17:10–5.
7. Schrier RW, Gross P, Gheorghiade M, et al. Tolvaptan, a selective oral vasopressin V2-receptor antagonist, for hyponatremia. N Engl J Med 2006;355:2099–112.
8. Ghali JK, Koren MJ, Taylor JR, et al. Efficacy and safety of oral conivaptan: A V1a/V2 vasopressin receptor antagonist, assessed in a randomized, placebo-controlled trial in patients with euvolemic or hypervolemic hyponatremia. J Clin Endocrinol Metab 2006;91:2145–52.
9. Zeltser D, Rosansky S, van Rensburg H, et al. Assessment of the efficacy and safety of intravenous conivaptan in euvolemic and hypervolemic hyponatremia. Am J Nephrol 2007;27(5):447–57.
10. Vaprisol [package insert]. Deerfield, IL: Astellas Pharma US, Inc; 2012.
11. Samsca [package insert]. Rockville, MD: Otsuka America Pharmaceutical, Inc; 2014.
12. Udelson JE, Smith WB, Hendrix GH, et al. Acute hemodynamic effects of conivaptan, a dual V1A and V2 vasopressin receptor antagonist, in patients with advanced heart failure. Circulation 2001;104:2417–23.
13. Goldsmith SR, Elkayam U, Haught WH, et al. Efficacy and safety of the vasopressin V1a/V2-receptor antagonist conivaptan in acute decompensated heart failure: a dose-ranging pilot study. J Card Fail 2008;14(8):641–7.
14. Costello-Boerrigter LC, Smith WB, Boerrigter G, et al. Vasopressin-2 receptor antagonist augments water excretion without changes in renal hemodynamics or sodium and potassium excretion in human heart failure. Am J Physiol Renal Physiol 2006;290:273–8.
15. Udelson JE, Orlandi C, Ouyang J, et al. Acute hemodynamic effects of tolvaptan, a vasopressin V2 receptor blocker, in patients with symptomatic heart failure and systolic dysfunction. J Am Coll Cardiol 2008;52(19):1540–5.
16. Gheorghiade M, Niazi I, Ouyang J, et al. Vasopressin V2-receptor blockade with tolvaptan in patients with chronic heart failure: results from a double-blind, randomized trial. Circulation 2003;107:2690–6.
17. Gheorghiade M, Cattis WA, O'Connor CM, et al. Effects of tolvaptan, a vasopressin antagonist, in

patients hospitalized with worsening heart failure, a randomized controlled trial (ACTIV in CHF). JAMA 2004;291(16):1963–71.

18. Udelson JE, McGrew FA, Flores E, et al. Multicenter, randomized, double-blind, placebo-controlled study on the effects of oral tolvaptan on left ventricular dilation and function in patients with heart failure and systolic dysfunction. J Am Coll Cardiol 2007;49(22):2151–9.

19. Gheorghiade M, Konstam M, Burnett J, et al. Short-term clinical effects of tolvaptan, an oral vaso-pressin antagonist, in patients hospitalized for heart failure: the EVEREST Clinical Status Trials. JAMA 2007;297(12):1332–43.

20. Konstam M, Gheorghiade M, Burnett J, et al. Effects of oral tolvaptan in patients hospitalized for worsening heart failure: the EVEREST Outcome Trial. JAMA 2007;297(12):1319–31.

21. Yancy CW, Jessup M, Bozkurt B, et al. 2013 ACCF/AHA Guideline for the management of heart failure. J Am Coll Cardiol 2013;62(16):e147–239.

22. Berl T, Quittnat-Pelletier F, Verbalis JG, et al. Oral tolvaptan is safe and effective in chronic hypona-tremia (SALTWATER). J Am Soc Nephrol 2010;21: 705–12.

23. Pang PS, Konstam MA, Krasa HB, et al. Effects of tolvaptan on dyspnea relief from the EVEREST tri-als. Eur Heart J 2009;30:2233–40.

24. Pang PS, Gheorghiade M, Dihu J, et al. Effects of tolvaptan on physician-assessed symptoms and signs in patients hospitalized with acute heart fail-ure syndromes: analysis from the EVEREST Trials. Am Heart J 2011;161:1067–72.

25. Rossi J, Bayram M, Udelson JE, et al. Improvement in hyponatremia during hospitalization for wors-ening heart failure is associated with improved out-comes: insights from the Acute and Chronic Therapeutic Impact of a Vasopressin Antagonist in Chronic Heart Failure (ACTIV in CHF) trial. Acute Card Care 2007;9:82–6.

26. Hauptman PJ, Burnett J, Gheorghiade M, et al. Clinical course of patients with hyponatremia and decompensated systolic heart failure and the effect of vasopressin receptor antagonism with tol-vaptan, from the EVEREST Trials. J Card Fail 2013; 19:390–7.

27. Felker GM, Duke University. Targeting acute conges-tion with tolvaptan in congestive heart failure (TAC-TICS-HF). 2014. Available at: http://clinicaltrials.gov/show/NCT01644331. Accessed May 16, 2014.

28. Konstam M, Cardiovascular Clinical Science Foun-dation. Randomized, double-blind, placebo-controlled study of the short term clinical effects of patients hospitalized for worsening heart failure with challenging volume management (SECRET in CHF). 2014. Available at: http://clinicaltrials.gov/show/NCT01584557. Accessed May 16, 2014.

29. Verbalis JG, Goldsmith SR, Greenberg A, et al. Diagnosis, evaluation, and treatment of hyponatre-mia: expert panel recommendations. Am J Med 2013;126:S8–42.

30. Goldsmith SR, Francis GS, Cowley AW Jr, et al. Increased plasma arginine vasopressin levels in patients with congestive heart failure. J Am Coll Cardiol 1983;1:1385–90.

31. Fonarow GC, Stough WG, Abraham WT, et al. Char-acteristics, treatments, and outcomes of patients with preserved systolic function hospitalized for heart failure – a report of the OPTIMIZE-HF registry. J Am Coll Cardiol 2007;50(8):768–77.

32. Felker GM, Benza RL, Chandler AB, et al. Heart failure etiology and response to milrinone in de-compensated heart failure: results from the OPTIME-CHF study. J Am Coll Cardiol 2003; 41(6):997–1003.

33. Francis GS, Benedict C, Johnstone DE, et al. Com-parison of neuroendocrine activation in patients with left ventricular dysfunction with and without congestive heart failure. A substudy of the Studies of Left Ventricular Dysfunction (SOLVD). Circulation 1990;82:1724–9.

34. Rosamond W, Flegal K, Furie K, et al. Heart dis-ease and stroke statistics – 2008 update: a report from the AHA Statistics Committee and Stroke Statistics Subcommittee. Circulation 2008;117: e25–146.

35. O'Connor CM, Abraham WT, Albert NM, et al. Pre-dictors of mortality after discharge in patients hos-pitalized with heart failure: an analysis from the organized program to initiate lifesaving treatment in hospitalized patients with heart failure (OPTI-MIZE-HF). Am Heart J 2008;156(4):662–73.

36. Adams KF, Fonarow GC, Emerman CL, et al. Char-acteristics and outcomes of patients hospitalized for heart failure in the United States: rationale, design, and preliminary observations from the first 100,000 cases in the Acute Decompensated Heart Failure National Registry (ADHERE). Am Heart J 2005;149:209–16.

37. Fonarow GC, Adams KF Jr, Abraham WT, et al. Risk stratification for in-hospital mortality in acutely decompensated heart failure: classification and regression tree analysis. JAMA 2005;293(5): 572–80.

38. Costanzo MR, Guglin ME, Saltzberg MT, et al. Ul-trafiltration versus intravenous diuretics for patients hospitalized for acute decompensated heart fail-ure. J Am Coll Cardiol 2007;49(6):675–83.

39. Young JB, Abraham WT, Stevenson LW, et al. Intra-venous nesiritide vs nitroglycerin for treatment of decompensated congestive heart failure: a ran-domized controlled trial, for the Vasodilation in the Management of Acute CHF (VMAC) investigators. JAMA 2002;287(12):1531–40.

40. Sackner-Bernstein JD, Kowalski M, Fox M, et al. Short-term risk of death after treatment with nesiritide for decompensated heart failure: a pooled analysis of randomized controlled trials. JAMA 2005;293(15):1900–5.

41. Greenberg A. Diuretic complications. Am J Med Sci 2000;319:10–24.

42. Weber KT. Furosemide in the long-term management of heart failure: the good, the bad, and the uncertain. J Am Coll Cardiol 2004;44(6): 1308–10.

43. Domanski M, Norman J, Pitt B, et al. Diuretic use, progressive heart failure, and death in patients in the Studies of Left Ventricular Dysfunction (SOLVD). J Am Coll Cardiol 2003;42(4):705–8.

44. Udelson JE, Bilsker M, Hauptman PJ, et al. A multicenter, randomized, double-blind, placebo-controlled study of tolvaptan monotherapy compared to furosemide and the combination of tolvaptan and furosemide in patients with heart failure and systolic dysfunction. J Card Fail 2011; 17(12):973–81.

45. Shoaf SE, Wang Z, Bricmont P, et al. Pharmacokinetics, pharmacodynamics, and safety of tolvaptan, a nonpeptide AVP antagonist, during ascending single-dose studies in healthy subjects. J Clin Pharmacol 2007;47(12):1498–507.

46. Kim S, Hasunuma T, Sato O, et al. Pharmacokinetic, pharmacodynamic and safety of tolvaptan – a novel, oral, selective non-peptide AVP V2-receptor antagonist: results of single- and multiple-dose studies in healthy Japanese male volunteers. Cardiovasc Drugs Ther 2011;25:S5–17.

47. Dasta JF, Chiong JR, Christian R, et al. Evaluation of costs associated with tolvaptan-mediated hospital length of stay reduction among US patients with the syndrome of inappropriate antidiuretic hormone secretion, based on SALT-1 and SALT-2 trials. Hosp Pract (1995) 2012;40:7–14.

48. Chiong JR, Kim S, Lin J, et al. Evaluation of costs associated with tolvaptan-mediated length-of-stay reduction among heart failure patients with hyponatremia in the US, based on the EVEREST trial. J Med Econ 2012;15:276–84.

49. Gheorghiade M, Pang S. Acute heart failure syndromes. J Am Coll Cardiol 2009;53(7):557–73.

50. Teerlink JR, Cotter G, Davison BA, et al. Serelaxin, recombinant human relaxin-2, for treatment of acute heart failure (RELAX-AHF): a randomized, placebo-controlled trial. Lancet 2013;381:29–39.

Lipid-Modifying Treatments for Heart Failure: Is Their Use Justified?

John G.F. Cleland, MD, PhD, FRCP, FESC[a],*,
Kate Hutchinson, MBChB[b], Pierpaolo Pellicori, MD[b],
Andrew Clark, MD, MA, FRCP[b]

KEYWORDS

- Fibrates • Polyunsaturated fatty acids • Statins • Heart failure

KEY POINTS

- Most patients with heart failure have atherosclerotic disease either as a cause of ventricular dysfunction or as a concomitant problem.
- Sudden death may be the most common presentation of myocardial infarction amongst patients with heart failure.
- Meta-analyses of trials of fibrates in cardiovascular disease identified no reduction in all-cause or cardiovascular mortality or heart failure events; there are no large trials of fibrates in patients with heart failure, but what evidence exists suggests no benefit.
- Meta-analyses of trials of polyunsaturated fatty acids in cardiovascular disease failed to show an effect on all-cause mortality but did suggest a small reduction in cardiac deaths (9% reduction in relative risk). There is equivocal evidence of benefit in patients with heart failure.
- Meta-analysis shows that statins reduce all-cause and cardiovascular mortality and heart failure events in patients with or at high risk of cardiovascular disease.

INTRODUCTION

There are theoretical arguments for and against lipid-modifying therapy for patients with heart failure but little conclusive clinical evidence that it provides substantial benefit or causes significant harm. However, one of the curses of modern therapeutics is polypharmacy. In a bygone era, the pharmacopoeia consisted of agents that were safe and ineffective (placebo) and those that might be effective but with varying degrees of toxicity.

Placebo does not prevent spontaneous recovery and may have psychological benefits and therefore often appears effective. The low benefit/risk ratio of interventions in this era gave rise to the old adage, "primum non nocere." Now that we have many more medicines, many of which are safe and effective, primum non nocere is no longer a tenable position, at least for serious diseases such as heart failure that rarely remit, because medicine practiced in this way is, paradoxically, quite likely to cause harm. A patient given too

Disclosure: Professor J.G.F. Cleland received honoraria for participation in the CORONA trial. No other relevant disclosures.
Professor J.G.F. Cleland is supported, in part, by the NIHR cardiovascular Biomedical Research Unit at the Royal Brompton and Harefield NHS Foundation Trust and Imperial College, London.
[a] National Heart & Lung Institute, Royal Brompton & Harefield Hospitals, Imperial College, London UB9 6JH, UK;
[b] Department of Cardiology, Hull York Medical School, Castle Hill Hospital, Kingston-upon-Hull HU6 5JQ, UK
* Corresponding author. Department of Cardiology, Harefield Hospital, Imperial College, Hill End Road, Harfield, Middlesex UB9 6JH, UK.
E-mail address: j.cleland@imperial.ac.uk

many medicines is likely not to take them all and may experience drug interactions. When faced with a plethora of choices, the motto of modern medicine for serious disease is "primum efficatum." Once an agent is shown to be effective, the penalty in terms of side effects, risk, and harm can be weighed. Of course, the power of placebo and concept of primum non nocere might still apply when the disease is likely to resolve spontaneously or causes little disability or when no effective treatments exist. Some medical disciplines are contaminated by agents upon which the medical community wastes huge amounts of money, for example, aspirin for long-term prophylaxis of cardiovascular disease,[1,2] most hypoglycemic agents for type-2 diabetes,[3] and vitamin and mineral supplements for osteoporosis.[4] The purpose of this report is to explore these issues with respect to lipid-modifying agents in patients with heart failure.

Most patients with heart failure have atherosclerosis, which is often the primary cause of their heart failure. Progression of atherosclerosis, which may impair blood flow to heart, brain, kidney, and skeletal muscle, and plaque rupture, leading to acute coronary and cerebrovascular syndromes, could be important pathways for the progression of heart failure, morbidity, and death.[5] Stabilizing plaque either by reducing its cholesterol content or by reducing inflammatory activity could reduce acute vascular events. Causing plaque to regress could reduce ischemia. Hyperlipidemia can also impair microvascular function that can be improved by lipid-lowering therapies.[6] Some authorities believe that all patients with heart failure due to left ventricular systolic dysfunction, regardless of its etiology, have myocardial ischemia, caused by epicardial coronary artery disease, microvascular dysfunction, elevated ventricular filling pressures, or potentially all three.[7]

Fatty acids are an important energy substrate for the myocardium but may be less efficient than glucose and lactate and may increase proton production, lowering cellular pH and impairing cell function. Diverting the myocardial energy substrate from lipids to carbohydrates might be beneficial.[8] Theoretically, lipid lowering might have beneficial effects on myocardial function. Lipid-modifying therapies may also have ancillary effects on inflammatory systems that might also improve myocardial function, encourage repair, reduce fibrosis, and increase electrical stability. However, higher plasma concentrations of arachidonic acid and some long-chain fatty acids, such as docosahexaenoic acid are associated with a lower incidence of heart failure.[9,10]

On the other hand, cholesterol decreases as heart failure progresses and a low cholesterol level is a bad prognostic sign in heart failure. This decrease may just reflect the metabolic stress of a patient who is in the process of dying from heart failure, but there is some concern that circulating lipid fractions may bind endotoxins absorbed from the gut.[11] Lowering cholesterol might impair this natural defense mechanism, cause cytokine activation, increase inflammation, and accelerate the progression of heart failure.[12] Moreover, statins can interfere with the synthesis of coenzyme Q10, an essential component of the mitochondrial respiratory chain.[13] Recent evidence suggests that coenzyme Q10 supplements may have a beneficial effect on prognosis in patients with heart failure.[14]

Lowering cholesterol might be both beneficial and harmful; in some patients the benefit will outweigh the harm; in others, harm and benefit will be similar, and the patient will derive no benefit. In some, harm may outweigh benefit. This article focuses on treatments designed to modify lipids; fibrates, statins and omega-3 fatty acids.

FIBRATES

There are no substantial randomized, controlled trials of fibrates in patients with heart failure. Node and colleagues[15] investigated the effects of bezafibrate on amino-terminal probrain natriuretic peptide (NT-proBNP) in 108 patients with New York Heart Association (NYHA) class III heart failure enrolled in the Bezafibrate Infarction Prevention study, a study of secondary prevention after a myocardial infarction. After 2 years of follow-up, plasma concentrations of NT-proBNP were similar in patients assigned to bezafibrate or placebo. In the overall population (with or without heart failure), the study was neutral.

Both the Veterans Affairs study of gemfibrozil[16] and the Action to Control Cardiovascular Risk in Diabetes (ACCORD) of fenofibrate[17] suggested fewer heart failure events in the actively managed group but no effect on all-cause or cardiovascular mortality. A meta-analysis of more than 45,000 patients in randomized, controlled trials of fibrates for the primary or secondary prevention of cardiovascular disease suggested no effect on all-cause or cardiovascular mortality or heart failure outcomes but a substantial effect on microvascular complications such as retinopathy among diabetic patients.[18]

There is little evidence to support the use of fibrates in patients with heart failure and insufficient trial evidence to confirm that they are either ineffective or safe.

OMEGA-3 FATTY ACIDS OR POLYUNSATURATED FATTY ACIDS

Overall, omega-3 fatty acids seem safe in patients with or at risk of cardiovascular disease, but the evidence of benefit is inconclusive. However, benefit may be modified depending on the country where the research was conducted. Most of the positive trials of omega-3 fatty acids come from Italy, a country where a lot of olive oil is used. Olive oil has commonly been used as the placebo intervention in trials of omega-3 fatty acids. However, in countries with low consumption of omega-3, olive oil may not be a placebo, although whether the dose of placebo olive oil is high enough to have a clinical effect is disputed.[19] In countries where olive oil consumption is high, a little extra olive oil might truly be a placebo, and the effect of omega-3 might become apparent.

The Gruppo Italiano per lo Studio della Sopravvivenza nell' Infarto miocardico (GISSI)-prevenzione trial[20] was a large (n = 11,324) randomized, double-blind trial comparing olive oil capsules with polyunsaturated fatty acids (PUFA) in patients with a recent myocardial infarction. The study found a reduction in mortality but not in nonfatal cardiovascular events. The major impact on mortality seemed to be caused by a reduction in sudden death, which many attributed to a reduction in ventricular arrhythmias but could also have been in part caused by a reduction in coronary events. A genuine reduction in coronary events combined with a reduction in prehospital arrhythmic mortality (patients who die before they reach the hospital cannot get a diagnosis) could account for the lack of effect on nonfatal events. The effect was greatest in patients with a reduced left ventricular ejection fraction, but perhaps only because this is a group with a higher rate of events. These observations triggered a second large study, GISSI-Heart Failure (HF) trial, which investigated the effects of rosuvastatin and PUFA on mortality.

GISSI-HF[21] included 6975 patients with NYHA class II to IV heart failure with or without a reduced left ventricular ejection fraction and randomized them, double-blind, to n-3 PUFA (1 g/d) or placebo. Patients not indicated for or already receiving a statin were then rerandomized to rosuvastatin or placebo (see later discussion). The coprimary outcome measures were all-cause mortality and the composite of death or admission to hospital for cardiovascular reasons. The median follow-up was 3.9 years (interquartile range, 3.0–4.5).

More than 40% of patients were older than 70 years, about half had known ischemic heart disease, and use of guideline-indicated treatment, apart perhaps from β-blockers, was good (**Table 1**).

Table 1
Patient characteristics in the GISSI-HF trial

	Placebo	n-3 PUFA
N	3481	3494
Age (y)	67	67
Age >70 y	43%	42%
Women	21%	22%
Ischemic heart disease	50%	49%
Dilated cardiomyopathy	28%	30%
NYHA II	63%	64%
Body mass index (kg/m²)	27	27
Systolic blood pressure (mm Hg)	126	126
Atrial fibrillation	16%	16%
Left ventricular ejection fraction >40%	9%	10%
Defibrillator	7%	7%
Diuretics	90%	90%
Angiotensin-converting enzyme inhibitor or angiotensin II receptor blockers	93%	94%
β-blockers	65%	65%
Spironolactone	40%	39%
Digoxin	37%	37%
Anti-coagulants	28%	29%
Statins	23%	22%

From Tavazzi L, Maggioni AP, Marchioli R, et al. Effect of n-3 polyunsaturated fatty acids in patients with chronic heart failure (the GISSI-HF trial): a randomised, double-blind, placebo-controlled trial. Lancet 2008;372(9645):1225; with permission.

Taking PUFA had no effect on heart rate or blood pressure and did not change total, high- or low-density lipoprotein cholesterol, although it did reduce triglycerides (P<.0001). A substudy suggested that PUFA could improve left ventricular ejection fraction, although the absolute difference from placebo was less than 1% at 3 years.[22]

Overall, 955 (27%) patients assigned to PUFA died, and 1014 (29%) of those assigned to placebo (olive oil) (adjusted hazard ratio [HR], 0.91; 95.5% confidence interval [CI], 0.833–0.998; P = .041), a result of borderline statistical significance (**Fig. 1**). Most deaths were cardiovascular (**Table 2**), but the reduction in cardiovascular death was not significant because of the slightly smaller number of events. Among causes of death, the reduction in sudden death was probably greatest (7.8% vs 8.7%). There were no subgroup interactions, but patients with left ventricular ejection fraction greater than 40% may have obtained less benefit.

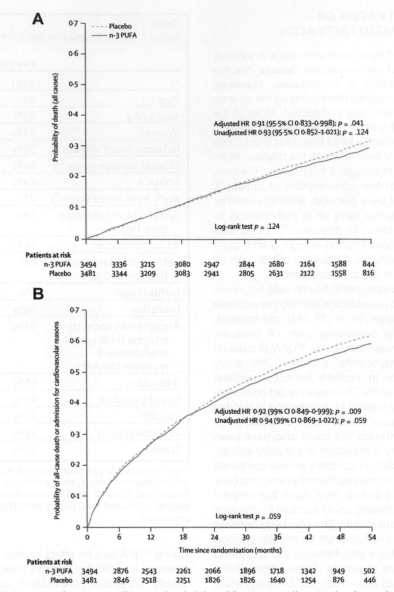

A

Probability of death (all causes)

Adjusted HR 0·91 (95·5% CI 0·833–0·998); p = .041
Unadjusted HR 0·93 (95·5% CI 0·852–1·021); p = .124

Log-rank test p = .124

Patients at risk

n-3 PUFA	3494	3336	3215	3080	2947	2844	2680	2164	1588	844
Placebo	3481	3344	3209	3083	2941	2805	2631	2122	1558	816

B

Probability of all-cause death or admission for cardiovascular reasons

Adjusted HR 0·92 (99% CI 0·849–0·999); p = .009
Unadjusted HR 0·94 (99% CI 0·869–1·022); p = .059

Log-rank test p = .059

Time since randomisation (months)

Patients at risk

n-3 PUFA	3494	2876	2543	2261	2066	1896	1718	1342	949	502
Placebo	3481	2846	2518	2251	1826	1826	1640	1254	876	446

Fig. 1. Kaplan-Meier curves for time to all-cause death (*A*) and for time to all-cause death or admission to hospital for cardiovascular reasons (*B*). (*From* Tavazzi L, Maggioni AP, Marchioli R, et al. Effect of n-3 polyunsaturated fatty acids in patients with chronic heart failure (the GISSI-HF trial): a randomised, double-blind, placebo-controlled trial. Lancet 2008;372(9645):1226; with permission.)

A cardiovascular admission or death occurred in 1981 (57%) patients assigned to PUFA and 2053 (59%) in those assigned to placebo (adjusted HR, 0.92; 99% CI, 0.849–0.999; P = .009). However, there was no reduction in hospitalization for heart failure (HR, 0.94).

In absolute terms, 56 patients needed to be treated for a median duration of 3.9 years to avoid one death or 44 to avoid the composite event. Similar numbers of patients withdrew from PUFA and placebo, mostly by choice rather than because of adverse reactions. However, a small trial of

patients with heart failure due to non-ischemic cardiomyopathy randomized 43 patients to placebo, 1 g/d or 4 g/d of PUFA. PUFA improved vascular function, markers of inflammation and left ventricular ejection fraction in a dose-dependent manner. Perhaps the dose of PUFA used in the studies conducted so far has been too low.[23]

These results should be interpreted in the wider context of trials of PUFA in populations at risk of heart failure such as those with or at high risk of cardiovascular disease. A meta-analysis including almost 70,000 patients identified no effect on

Table 2
Causes of death

	n-3 PUFA (N = 3494) (%)	Placebo (N = 3481) (%)
Total mortality	955 (27.3)	1014 (29.1)
Acute myocardial infarction	20 (0.6)	25 (0.7)
Worsening heart failure	319 (9.1)	332 (9.5)
Presumed arrhythmic	274 (7.8)	304 (8.7)
Stroke	50 (1.4)	44 (1.3)
Other cardiovascular reasons	49 (1.4)	60 (1.7)
Neoplasia	107 (3.1)	112 (3.2)
Other noncardiovascular reasons	97 (2.8)	102 (2.9)
Not known	39(1.1)	35 (1.0)

From Tavazzi L, Maggioni AP, Marchioli R, et al. Effect of n-3 polyunsaturated fatty acids in patients with chronic heart failure (the GISSI-HF trial): a randomised, double-blind, placebo-controlled trial. Lancet 2008;372(9645):1227; with permission.

all-cause mortality but suggested a small reduction (HR, 0.91; 95% CI, 0.85–0.98) in cardiac deaths. However, in a subgroup of trials conducted in patients with implanted defibrillators, a substantial effect on all-cause mortality (HR, 0.69; 95% CI, 0.39–1.23) could not be excluded.[24]

Current guidelines from the European Society of Cardiology give a class IIb, level of evidence B recommendation for PUFA,[25] a fairly weak recommendation that seems warranted by the totality of the evidence. Guidelines from the American Heart Association/American College of Cardiology give a stronger recommendation: class IIa, level of evidence B.[26]

STATINS (3-HYDROXY-3-METHYLGLUTARYL-COENZYME-A REDUCTASE INHIBITORS)

Many have been intrigued by the rather low incidence of myocardial infarction in clinical trials of heart failure despite the high prevalence of ischemic heart disease.[5,27,28] This low incidence could be because coronary events are uncommon and contribute little to the progression of disease or mortality. Alternatively, we know that many patients have coronary events but do not have typical symptoms. Cardiac denervation as a consequence of diabetes or previous cardiac damage may modify symptoms and might account for why many patients with worsening heart failure have elevated biomarkers of cardiac damage in the absence of classical symptoms of myocardial ischemia or infarction. Another important reason why the incidence of myocardial infarction may be so low is that patients with preexisting cardiac dysfunction may be much more likely to die suddenly of arrhythmias or shock before they can get medical attention and a diagnosis of infarction.[29] Thus, statins could reduce further silent cardiac

damage as well as overt vascular events and sudden death. Statins might also have other effects, such as improving microvascular function or reducing myocardial inflammation.[12,30]

Observational studies suggest that patients treated with statins have a better outcome than those who are not, after adjusting for measured confounders such as age and ischemic heart disease.[31–34] However, many unmeasured confounders make such adjusted observational analyses unreliable. The effect seemed to be mainly on sudden death, although it is unclear whether this is vascular or arrhythmic sudden death. Patients without known coronary artery disease also seemed to benefit.[33]

Smaller randomized, controlled trials suggested that statins could reduce cholesterol and some markers of inflammation such as soluble tumor necrosis factor receptor-1 and C-reactive protein but not others such as interleukin-6.[35,36] Atorvastatin also reduced endothelin-1 but not brain natriuretic peptide.[35] Effects on ventricular function have been variable,[22,36–38] with some randomized studies reporting improvement even in patients without coronary disease[36] and reductions in natriuretic peptides.[37] Some small trials even suggested a reduction in sudden death and overall mortality.[39]

The next level of evidence comes from subgroup analyses of large clinical trials in populations that contained some patients with heart failure. The Treating to New Targets (TNT) Study compared two doses of atorvastatin, 80 mg/d and 10 mg/d, in patients with coronary disease.[40] Patients had to have stable coronary disease and a left ventricular ejection fraction greater than 30%. Hospitalizations for heart failure in the overall population (10,001) were reduced from 3.3% to 2.4% (HR, 0.74; 95% CI, 0.59–0.94; *P*<.0116) with higher-dose statin over a median follow-up of 4.9 years. The rate of hospitalization for heart failure seems low in both arms, suggesting that many cases were missed. The higher the baseline cholesterol, the greater was the risk of a heart failure event and the greater the difference in effect between doses. Of 10,001 patients enrolled, only 7.8% had some degree of heart failure at baseline, but it must have been very mild, as only about 50% of them were prescribed a diuretic. The effect of the higher dose of atorvastatin on hospitalization for heart failure was more marked in patients with a history of heart failure at baseline: 17.3% versus 10.6% in the 10-mg and 80-mg arms, respectively (HR, 0.59; 95% CI, 0.4–0.88; P<.009).

Finally, three substantial studies, two with rosuvastatin, a hydrophilic agent, and one with pitavastatin, a lipophilic agent, have been conducted; all were neutral for their primary endpoint.

GISSI-HF

The GISSI-HF trial investigated the safety and efficacy of rosuvastatin 10 mg/d in 4574 patients with

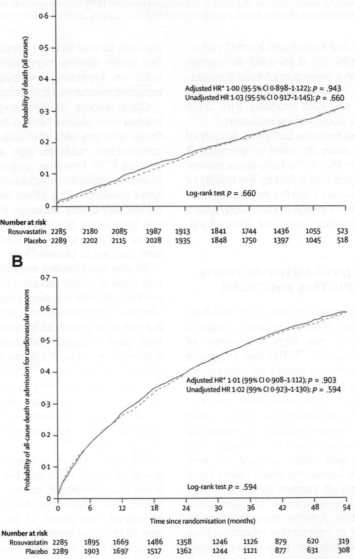

Fig. 2. Kaplan-Meier curves for time to all-cause death (A) and for time to all-cause death or admission for cardiovascular reasons (B). (*From* Gissi-HF Investigators, Tavazzi L, Maggioni AP, et al. Effect of rosuvastatin in patients with chronic heart failure (the GISSI-HF trial): a randomised, double-blind, placebo-controlled trial. Lancet 2008;372(9645):1234; with permission.)

symptomatic heart failure, irrespective of age or left ventricular ejection fraction and included patients both with and without ischemic heart disease. Patients with a recent vascular event or with a serum creatinine level greater than 221 μmol/L were excluded. The coprimary outcome measures were all-cause mortality and the composite of death or admission to hospital for cardiovascular reasons. The median follow-up was 3.9 years (interquartile range, 3.0–4.4).

More than 40% of patients were older than 70 years, about half had known ischemic heart disease, and use of guideline-indicated treatment, apart perhaps from β-blockers (63%), was good. Taking rosuvastatin reduced C-reactive protein and low-density lipoprotein cholesterol levels (from 3.16 mmol/L to 2.15 mmol/L; P<.0001)[41] but had no effect on high-density lipoprotein cholesterol or left ventricular ejection fraction.[22]

There were 657 (29%) deaths in patients assigned to rosuvastatin (29%) compared with 644 (28%) in those assigned to placebo (P = .76) (**Fig. 2**). The composite outcome of death or admission to the hospital for cardiovascular reasons occurred in 1305 (57%) patients assigned to rosuvastatin and 1283 (56%) assigned to placebo. All other secondary endpoints were neutral as were all subgroup analyses. Similar numbers of patients stopped rosuvastatin and placebo.

CORONA

The CORONA (Controlled rosuvastatin multinational study in heart failure) trial[42] investigated the safety and efficacy of rosuvastatin 10 mg/d in 5011 patients older than 60 years with symptomatic heart failure and at least some evidence of ischemic heart disease. Left ventricular ejection fraction had to be less than 40% unless the patient was in NYHA class II, in which case it had to be less than 35%. Patients with a recent vascular event or with a serum creatinine level greater than 221 μmol/L were excluded. The primary outcome was nonfatal myocardial infarction or stroke or cardiovascular death. The median follow-up was 33 months (**Table 3**).

More than 40% of patients were aged older than 75 years, and most were on full contemporary guideline-indicated therapy. Taking rosuvastatin reduced C-reactive protein, triglyceride, and low-density lipoprotein cholesterol levels (from 3.54 mmol/L to 1.96 mmol/L; P<.0001) and increased levels of high-density lipoprotein cholesterol.

The primary composite endpoint occurred in 732 (29%) patients assigned to placebo and 692

Table 3
Patient characteristics in the CORONA trial

	Placebo	Rosuvastatin
N	2497	2514
Age (y)	73	73
Age >75 y	41%	41%
Women	24%	24%
NYHA II	37%	37%
Body mass index (kg/m²)	27	27
Systolic blood pressure (mm Hg)	129	129
Atrial fibrillation	23%	24%
Defibrillator	3%	3%
Diuretics	88% (75% loop)	89% (76% loop)
Angiotensin-converting enzyme inhibitor or angiotensin II receptor blockers	92%	91%
β-blockers	75%	75%
Aldosterone antagonist	39%	39%
Digoxin	32%	34%
Anticoagulants	34%	36%
NT-proBNP (ng/L)	1404 (600–2960)	1522 (626–3247)
Total cholesterol	5.4	5.4
Low-density lipoprotein cholesterol	3.6	3.5

Data from Kjekshus J, Apetrei E, Barrios V, et al. Rosuvastatin in older patients with systolic heart failure. N Engl J Med 2007;357(22):2250–1; with permission.

(28%) assigned to rosuvastatin (HR, 0.92; 95% CI, 0.83–1.02; P = .12), and all-cause mortality was 759 (30%) and 728 (29%), respectively (HR, 0.95; 95% CI, 0.86–1.05; P = 0.31) (**Fig. 3**). A non-prespecified outcome of nonfatal or fatal myocardial infarction or stroke was slightly lower in patients assigned to rosuvastatin (HR, 0.84; 95% CI, 0.70–1.00; P = .05). There were fewer hospitalizations for cardiovascular causes, including worsening heart failure, in the rosuvastatin group (2193) than the placebo group (2564; P<.001; see **Fig. 3**). Withdrawals and adverse effects were similar in each group.

A prespecified subgroup analysis identified little heterogeneity in the results. However, when results were analyzed by tercile of NT-proBNP, patients in the lowest third had the lowest rate of events but the greatest reduction in risk with rosuvastatin. A subsequent analysis, in which the data were combined with those from the Heart Protection study (N = 20,536), comparing simvastatin with placebo in a broad range of older patients at high risk of vascular disease, suggested that the greatest relative benefit of statins was among those with the lowest NT-proBNP.[43] As NT-proBNP increased, the population risk increased, but the relative benefit of simvastatin decreased. Combining the data from CORONA completed the picture, predicting no effect of statins on major vascular events or mortality when values exceeded approximately 800 ng/L (the upper limit of the lower tertile of values in CORONA; **Fig. 4**). However, a reduction in hospitalizations was still observed even with higher NT-proBNP values. An analysis of serum coenzyme Q10 concentrations found that lower levels were associated with a poorer prognosis, but this was explained by greater age and frailty of the patients. Rosuvastatin reduced serum coenzyme Q10, but its effects were similar regardless of baseline or change in serum levels of Q10.[13]

PEARL

The PEARL (Pitavastatin Heart Failure) study enrolled 574 patients with chronic heart failure and randomized them to placebo or pitavsatatin, a lipophilic statin. Pitavastatin failed to reduce

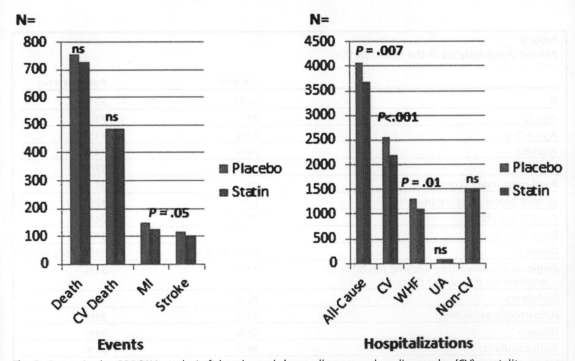

Fig. 3. Events in the CORONA study. Left hand panel shows all-cause and cardiovascular (CV) mortality, myocardial infarction, and stroke (P = .05 for the difference between placebo and rosuvastatin on myocardial infarction and stroke combined). Right hand panel shows the number of hospitalization events; all-cause, cardiovascular, worsening heart failure (WHF), unstable angina (UA), and noncardiovascular. (*From* Kjekshus J, Apetrei E, Barrios V, et al. Rosuvastatin in older patients with systolic heart failure. N Engl J Med 2007;357(22):2248–61; with permission.)

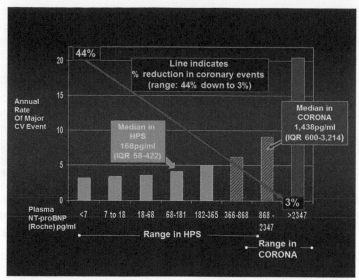

Fig. 4. Relationship between NT-proBNP and major CV events in the Heart Protection Study and CORONA. (*From* Cleland JG, Squire I, Ng L. Interpretation of amino-terminal pro-brain natriuretic peptide levels in the HPS and the CORONA study. J Am Coll Cardiol 2008;52(13):1104; with permission.)

the primary composite outcome (cardiac death or hospitalization for worsening heart failure - hazard ratio 0.92, 95% CI 0.63–1.35, *P* = 0.672). However, a strong interaction between assigned treatment and left ventricular ejection fraction was observed (*P* = 0.004); those with an ejection fraction ≥30% gained substantial benefit (hazard ratio 0.53, 95% CI 0.31–0.90, *P* = 0.018) with

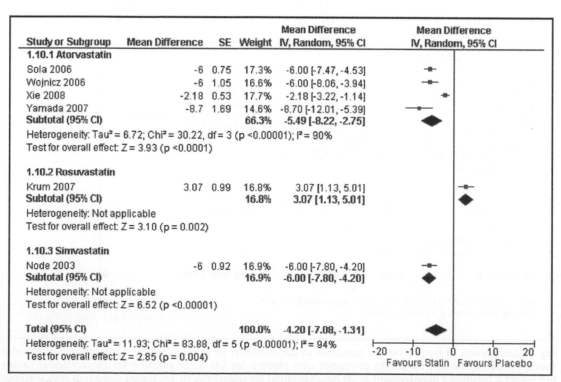

Fig. 5. Effect of statins on left ventricular ejection fraction. Since this report, GISS-HF also reported no difference between rosuvastatin and placebo. (*From* Lipinski MJ, Cauthen CA, Biondi-Zoccai GG, et al. Meta-analysis of randomized controlled trials of statins versus placebo in patients with heart failure. Am J Cardiol 2009;104(12):1713; with permission.)

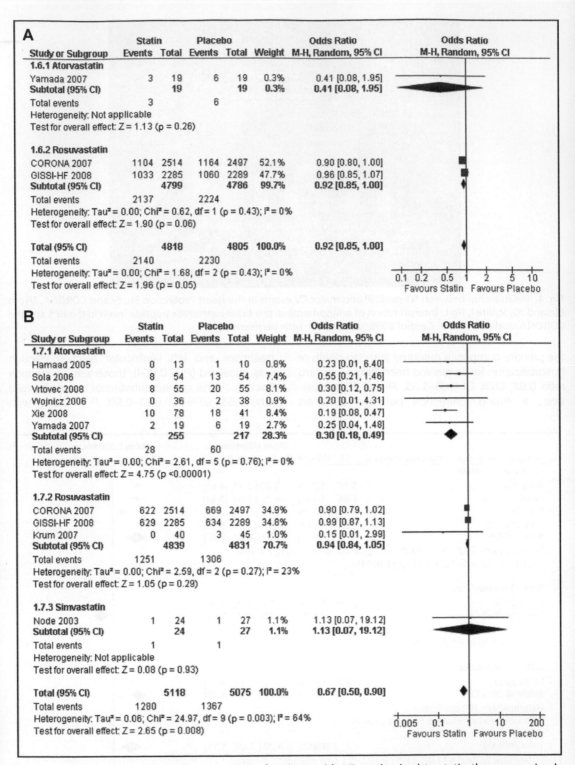

Fig. 6. Comparison of hospitalization outcomes of patients with HF randomized to statin therapy or placebo found no overall benefit for statins compared with placebo for (*A*) hospitalization for cardiovascular causes but found a significant improvement in (*B*) hospitalization for worsening HF for statins compared with placebo. (*From* Lipinski MJ, Cauthen CA, Biondi-Zoccai GG, et al. Meta-analysis of randomized controlled trials of statins versus placebo in patients with heart failure. Am J Cardiol 2009;104(12):1712; with permission.)

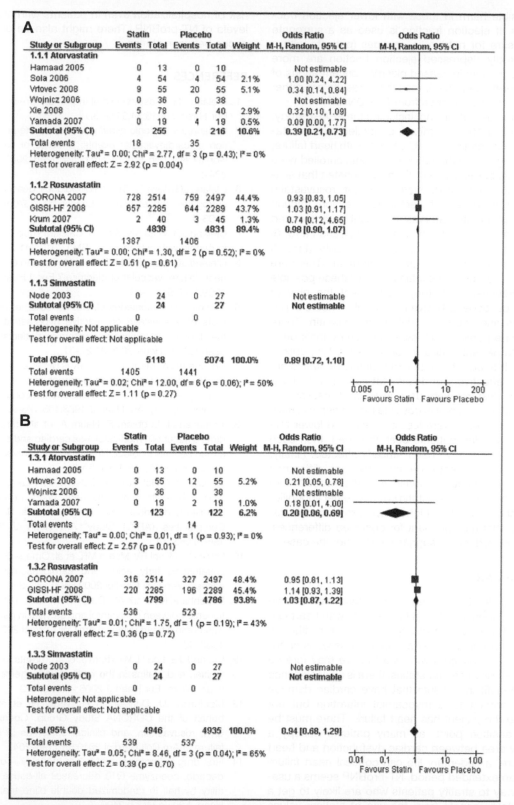

Fig. 7. Randomized, controlled trials of statins reporting all-cause mortality (*A*) or sudden death (*B*) in patients with heart failure. (*From* Lipinski MJ, Cauthen CA, Biondi-Zoccai GG, et al. Meta-analysis of randomized controlled trials of statins versus placebo in patients with heart failure. Am J Cardiol 2009;104(12):1711; with permission.)

possible harm in those with lower ejection fractions. If ejection fraction is used as a surrogate measure for natriuretic peptides (patients with a markedly depressed ejection fraction are more likely to have increased plasma concentrations of natriuretic peptides), then these results are rather consistent with those from CORONA.[44]

A meta-analysis, not including the PEARL study, identified 10 randomized, controlled trials of statins that enrolled 10,192 patients with heart failure, although more than 95% of patients enrolled were in trials of rosuvastatin.[45] This suggested that simvastatin and atorvastatin but not rosuvastatin might improve left ventricular ejection fraction (**Fig. 5**) and that atorvastatin might be associated with a greater reduction in hospitalization (**Fig. 6**) and a reduction in all-cause mortality (**Fig. 7**) driven by a reduction in sudden death. There are at least 5 possible explanations for these possible differences. First, they may reflect the play of chance, especially given the small numbers of patients and events in trials of atorvastatin. There may be publication bias; small neutral trials often fail to get submitted for or accepted for publication. It is possible that larger doses of statins are more effective, but doses that had similar effects on cholesterol were used in trials of rosuvastatin and atorvastatin. It is possible that patients in trials of atorvastatin were less sick and had lower NT-proBNP. Had patients been matched, then each agent might have been similarly affected. Finally, there might really be an important difference between agents. Atorvastatin and simvastatin are lipophilic but rosuvastatin is not. Greater lipophilicity should lead to higher myocardial concentrations that may account for observed differences. The PEARL study suggests this is not the case.

SUMMARY

So far, lipid-modifying interventions have shown little evidence of benefit in patients with heart failure. The evidence to support the use of fibrates and PUFA in the general population is weak or absent, and patients with heart failure may fare no better. However, for statins, there is clear evidence of benefit in patients that have cardiac damage subsequent to a myocardial infarction but not once the patient has heart failure. There must be a transition point, as many patients occupy a gray area between cardiac dysfunction and heart failure; a sedentary life can conceal heart failure for an extended period. NT-proBNP seems a useful way to stratify patients who are likely to get a mortality benefit from the use of statins; values less than 800 ng/L are associated with benefit. However, statins seem safe and may reduce the

risk of hospitalization even in patients with higher levels of NT-proBNP. There might also be differences between statins.

REFERENCES

1. Cleland JG. Is aspirin useful in primary prevention? Eur Heart J 2013;34:3412–8.
2. Cleland JG. Chronic aspirin therapy for the prevention of cardiovascular events: a waste of time or worse? Nat Clin Pract Cardiovasc Med 2006;3(5): 234–5.
3. Cleland JG, Atkin SL. Thiazolidinediones, deadly sins, surrogates and elephants. Lancet 2007;370(9593): 1103–4.
4. Cleland JG, Witte KK, Steel S. Calcium supplements in people with osteoporosis. BMJ 2010;341:c3856.
5. Cleland JG, Massie BM, Packer M. Sudden death in heart failure: vascular or electrical? Eur J Heart Fail 1999;1:41–5.
6. Tousoulis D, Antoniades C, Bosinakou E, et al. Effects of atorvastatin on reactive hyperaemia and the thrombosis–fibrinolysis system in patients with heart failure. Heart 2005;91:27–31.
7. Unverferth DV, Magorien RD, Lewis RP, et al. The role of subendocardial ischemia in perpetuating myocardial failure in patients with non-ischemic congestive cardiomyopathy. Am Heart J 1983;105:176–9.
8. Tuunanen H, Engblom E, Naum A, et al. Trimetazidine, a metabolic modulator, has cardiac and extracardiac benefits in idiopathic dilated cardiomyopathy. Circulation 2008;118(12):1250–8.
9. Yamagishi K, Nettleton JA, Folsom AR. Plasma fatty acid composition and incident heart failure in middle-aged adults: the Atherosclerosis Risk in Communities (ARIC) Study. Am Heart J 2008; 156(5):965–74.
10. Lavie CJ, Milani RV, Mehra MR, et al. Omega-3 polyunsaturated fatty acids and cardiovascular diseases. J Am Coll Cardiol 2009;54(7):585–94.
11. Rauchhaus M, Clark AL, Doehner W, et al. The relationship between cholesterol and survival in patients with chronic heart failure. J Am Coll Cardiol 2003;42: 1933–40.
12. Cleland JG, Loh H, Windram J, et al. Threats, opportunities and statins in the modern management of heart failure. Eur Heart J 2006;27(6):641–3.
13. McMurray JJ, Dunselman P, Wedel H, et al, on behalf of the CORONA Study Group. Coenzyme Q10, rosuvastatin, and clinical outcomes in heart failure. J Am Coll Cardiol 2010;56:1196–204.
14. First drug to improve heart failure mortality in over a decade: coenzyme Q10 decreases all-cause mortality by half in randomized double blind trial. Eur Heart J 2013;34(32):2496–7.
15. Node K, Inoue T, Boyko V, et al. Long-term effects of peroxisome proliferator-activated receptor ligand

bezafibrate on N-terminal pro-B type natriuretic peptide in patients with advanced functional capacity impairment. Cardiovasc Diabetol 2009;8:5.

16. Rubins HB, Robins SJ, Collins D, et al. Gemfibrozil for the secondary prevention of coronary heart disease in men with low levels of high-density lipoprotein cholesterol. Veterans Affairs High-Density Lipoprotein Cholesterol Intervention Trial Study Group. N Engl J Med 1999;341(6):410–8.

17. Ginsberg HN, Elam MB, Lovato LC, et al. Effects of combination lipid therapy in type 2 diabetes mellitus. N Engl J Med 2010;362(17):1563–74.

18. Jun M, Foote C, Lv J, et al. Effects of fibrates on cardiovascular outcomes: a systematic review and meta-analysis. Lancet 2010;375(9729):1875–84.

19. Cleland JG, Joseph A, Pellicori P. Fish oil vs olive oil for postoperative atrial fibrillation. JAMA 2013; 309(9):871.

20. Dietary supplementation with n-3 polyunsaturated fatty acids and vitamin E after myocardial infarction: results of the GISSI-Prevenzione trial. Gruppo Italiano per lo Studio della Sopravvivenza nell'Infarto miocardico. Lancet 1999;354(9177):447–55.

21. Tavazzi L, Maggioni AP, Marchioli R, et al. Effect of n-3 polyunsaturated fatty acids in patients with chronic heart failure (the GISSI-HF trial): a randomised, double-blind, placebo-controlled trial. Lancet 2008; 372(9645):1223–30.

22. Ghio S, Scelsi L, Latini R, et al. Effects of n-3 polyunsaturated fatty acids and of rosuvastatin on left ventricular function in chronic heart failure: a substudy of GISSI-HF trial. Eur J Heart Fail 2010;12(12):1345–53.

23. Moertl D, Hammer A, Steiner S, et al. Dose-dependent effects of omega-3-polyunsaturated fatty acids on systolic left ventricular function, endothelial function, and markers of inflammation in chronic heart failure of nonischemic origin: A double-blind, placebo-controlled, 3-arm study. Am Heart J 2011; 161(5):915.e1–9.

24. Rizos EC, Ntzani EE, Bika E, et al. Association between omega-3 fatty acid supplementation and risk of major cardiovascular disease events: a systematic review and meta-analysis. JAMA 2012;308(10): 1024–33.

25. McMurray JJ, Adamopoulos S, Anker SD, et al. ESC guidelines for the diagnosis and treatment of acute and chronic heart failure 2012: the task force for the diagnosis and treatment of acute and chronic heart failure 2012 of the European Society of Cardiology. Developed in collaboration with the Heart Failure Association (HFA) of the ESC. Eur J Heart Fail 2012;14:803–69.

26. Yancy CW, Jessup M, Bozkurt B, et al. 2013 ACCF/AHA guideline for the management of heart failure: a report of the American College of Cardiology Foundation/American Heart Association task force on practice guidelines. J Am Coll Cardiol 2013;62(16):e147–239.

27. Cleland JG, Thygesen K, Uretsky BF, et al. Cardiovascular critical event pathways for the progression of heart failure. A report from the ATLAS study. Eur Heart J 2001;22:1601–12.

28. Khand AU, Gemmell I, Rankin AC, et al. Clinical events leading to the progression of heart failure: insights from a national database of hospital discharges. Eur Heart J 2001;22:153–64.

29. Uretsky B, Thygesen K, Armstrong PW, et al. Acute coronary findings at autopsy in heart failure patients with sudden death: Results from the assessment of treatment with lisinopril and survival study (ATLAS) trial. Circulation 2000;102:611–6.

30. Windram J, Loh PH, Rigby AS, et al. Relationship of high-sensitivity C-reactive protein to prognosis and other prognostic markers in outpatients with heart failure. Am Heart J 2007;153(6):1048–55.

31. Krum H, Latini R, Maggioni AP, et al. Statins and symptomatic chronic systolic heart failure: a post-hoc analysis of 5010 patients enrolled in Val-HeFT. Int J Cardiol 2007;119(1):48–53.

32. Mozaffarian D, Nye R, Levy WC. Statin therapy is associated with lower mortality among patients with severe heart failure. Am J Cardiol 2004;93:1124–9.

33. Go AS, Lee WY, Yang J, et al. Statin therapy and risks for death and hospitalization in chronic heart failure. JAMA 2006;296(17):2105–11.

34. Huan LP, Windram JD, Tin L, et al. The effects of initiation or continuation of statin therapy on cholesterol level and all-cause mortality after the diagnosis of left ventricular systolic dysfunction. Am Heart J 2007;153(4):537–44.

35. Mozaffarian D, Minami E, Letterer RA, et al. The effects of atorvastatin (10 mg) on systemic inflammation in heart failure. Am J Cardiol 2005;96(12):1699–704.

36. Sola S, Mir MQ, Lerakis S, et al. Atorvastatin improves left ventricular systolic function and serum markers of inflammation in nonischemic heart failure. J Am Coll Cardiol 2006;47(2):332–7.

37. Yamada T, Node K, Mine T, et al. Long-term effect of atorvastatin on neurohumoral activation and cardiac function in patients with chronic heart failure: a prospective randomized controlled study. Am Heart J 2007;153(6):1055–8.

38. Wojnicz R, Wilczek K, Nowalany-Kozielska E, et al. Usefulness of atorvastatin in patients with heart failure due to inflammatory dilated cardiomyopathy and elevated cholesterol levels. Am J Cardiol 2006; 97(6):899–904.

39. Vrtovec B, Okrajsek R, Golicnik A, et al. Atorvastatin therapy may reduce the incidence of sudden cardiac death in patients with advanced chronic heart failure. J Card Fail 2008;14(2):140–4.

40. Khush KK, Waters DD, Bittner V, et al. Effect of high-dose atorvastatin on hospitalizations for heart failure: subgroup analysis of the Treating to New Targets (TNT) study. Circulation 2007;115(5):576–83.

41. Gissi-HF Investigators, Tavazzi L, Maggioni AP, et al. Effect of rosuvastatin in patients with chronic heart failure (the GISSI-HF trial): a randomised, double-blind, placebo-controlled trial. Lancet 2008;372(9645): 1231–9.

42. Kjekshus J, Apetrei E, Barrios V, et al, CORONA Group. Rosuvastatin in older patients with systolic heart failure. N Engl J Med 2007;357(22):2248–61.

43. Cleland JG, Squire I, Ng L. Interpretation of amino-terminal pro-brain natriuretic peptide levels in the

HPS and the CORONA study. J Am Coll Cardiol 2008;52(13):1104–5.

44. Takano H, Mizuma H, Kuwabara Y, et al. Effects of Pitavastatin in Japanese Patients With Chronic Heart Failure: the Pitavastatin Heart Failure Study (PEARL Study). Circ J 2013;77(4):917–25.

45. Lipinski MJ, Cauthen CA, Biondi-Zoccai GG, et al. Meta-analysis of randomized controlled trials of statins versus placebo in patients with heart failure. Am J Cardiol 2009;104(12):1708–16.

Current Approaches to Antiarrhythmic Therapy in Heart Failure

Lisa J. Rose-Jones, MD[a,*], Weeranun D. Bode, MD[b],
Anil K. Gehi, MD[c]

KEYWORDS

- Congestive heart failure • Antiarrhythmics • Atrial fibrillation • Rhythm control
- Ventricular tachycardia • Electrical storm • ICD shocks

KEY POINTS

- Atrial fibrillation (AF) is exceedingly common in patients with heart failure (HF), as they share common risk factors.
- Rate control is the cornerstone of treatment for AF in patients with HF; however, restoration of sinus rhythm should be considered when more than minimal symptoms are present.
- Although implantable cardioverter defibrillators (ICDs) protect against sudden cardiac arrest in patients with HF, many will present with ventricular tachycardia (VT) or ICD shocks.
- Antiarrhythmic drug therapy beyond beta-blocker therapy remains fundamental to the termination of acute VT and the prevention of ICD shocks.

INTRODUCTION

Antiarrhythmic drug therapy is used for 3 major purposes in patients with congestive heart failure (HF): maintenance of sinus rhythm (SR) in those with atrial fibrillation (AF), acute treatment of ventricular tachycardia (VT), and prevention of implantable cardioverter defibrillator (ICD) shocks. Management of arrhythmias in patients with HF requires nuance on the part of the provider. The efficacy of antiarrhythmic drugs must be balanced against its potential side effects and alternate therapies. Nevertheless, antiarrhythmic drug therapy retains a significant role in the chronic management of patients with HF.

SUPRAVENTRICULAR ARRHYTHMIA

Supraventricular tachycardia (SVT) is an arrhythmia that originates from the atria. The most common of these is AF. Other SVTs include atrial flutter, atrioventricular nodal reentrant tachycardia (AVNRT), atrioventricular reentrant tachycardia (AVRT), and atrial tachycardia. Typical atrial flutter (AFL), AVNRT, and AVRT are best treated with catheter ablation due to its high success rate and low risk of complications.[1] However, AF, atypical atrial flutter, and certain forms of atrial tachycardia often are treated first with medical therapy in the form of an antiarrhythmic drug. This review focuses on AF, the most prevalent atrial arrhythmia, which often is treated with antiarrhythmic drug therapy.

AF: EPIDEMIOLOGY AND PATHOPHYSIOLOGY

AF is the most common arrhythmia and is increasing in prevalence.[2] Current estimates are that AF affects 2.2 million people in the United States and it is projected that number will be approximately 15 million

[a] Advanced Heart Failure & Pulmonary Hypertension, UNC Heart & Vascular Center, 6th Floor, Burnett-Womack Building, 160 Dental Circle, CB#7075, Chapel Hill, NC 27599, USA; [b] Clinical Fellow, UNC Heart & Vascular Center, 6th Floor, Burnett-Womack Building, 160 Dental Circle, CB#7075, Chapel Hill, NC 27599, USA; [c] Electrophysiology, UNC Heart & Vascular Center, 6th Floor, Burnett-Womack Building, 160 Dental Circle, CB#7075, Chapel Hill, NC 27599, USA
* Corresponding author.
E-mail address: Lisa_rose-jones@med.unc.edu

Heart Failure Clin 10 (2014) 635–652
http://dx.doi.org/10.1016/j.hfc.2014.07.010
1551-7136/14/$ – see front matter © 2014 Elsevier Inc. All rights reserved.

by 2050.[3] HF is one of the leading causes of death worldwide and its incidence is also increasing.[4,5] These companion epidemics have accelerated the need for management options for AF in this population.

Chronic HF results in structural remodeling that creates an ideal substrate for atrial fibrillation. There is a complex interplay among ultrastructural, electrophysiologic, and neurohormonal changes that promote the coexistence of AF in HF (Fig. 1)[6–9]:

- Persistent left atrial hypertension from poor left ventricular (LV) chamber compliance and function promotes interstitial fibrosis and decreased gap junction surface area
- Structural myocyte changes lead to a reduction of repolarizing potassium currents and

consequently abnormal intracellular calcium handling
- A decline in electrical coupling between neighboring myocytes slows conduction within the myocardium
- Baseline pathophysiological activation of the sympathetic system
- HF medications may perturb electrolytes, which can influence further susceptibility to a proarrhythmic state

HF and AF share several risk factors, including coronary artery disease, diabetes mellitus, hypertension, obesity, and obstructive sleep apnea.[10] These contributing factors lead to a high prevalence of AF in HF, affecting 30% of all individuals with HF, including those with reduced or preserved ejection fraction.[11,12] In addition, there is

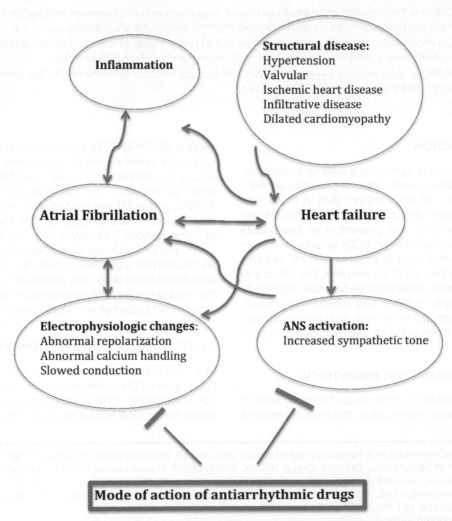

Fig. 1. There is a complex relationship between the multiple factors that promote the coexistence of AF in HF; antiarrhythmics can be used to target electrophysiologic changes and abnormal autonomics which promote AF. ANS, autonomic nervous system.

a direct relationship between the prevalence of AF and worsening HF class.[13] Thus, the treatment of AF in patients with HF may be an important step to prevent further worsening of HF symptoms leading to hospitalization or mortality.

Although many studies have shown that the presence of AF in patients with HF is associated with an adverse prognosis, it remains unclear whether targeting AF with a view to maintaining SR improves outcomes.[11,14–17]

ACUTE MANAGEMENT OF AF IN PATIENTS WITH HF

One-third of patients with HF with an acute exacerbation present in AF with rapid ventricular response, potentially precipitating an acute HF exacerbation.[14,18] Several aspects to the therapy of acute AF need to be considered:

- Atrioventricular (AV) nodal blockade has become the mainstay of therapy for rate control, as it limits how quickly rapid fibrillatory waves reach the ventricle
- Beta-adrenergic receptor blockers (beta-blockers), nondihydropyridine calcium channel blockers (CCBs), and digitalis glycosides prolong the refractoriness of the AV node and can be used for reducing ventricular rate[19]
- Analysis from the AFFIRM study demonstrated that beta-blockers were more effective than CCBs in the acute setting for rate control (70% vs 54%, respectively)[20]
- Additionally, CCBs have negative inotropic effect, and should be avoided in those with significant LV dysfunction
- Digitalis has a slower onset of action and is relatively ineffective in higher adrenergic states; should be avoided for acute rate control[2]
- Direct current cardioversion (DCCV) is the most effective method for conversion to SR, but clinicians must consider the risk of sedation (ie, stable patient with HF can be susceptible to drops in blood pressure)[21]
- Transesophageal echocardiogram (TEE) is necessary to rule out left atrial clot before DCCV if the AF episode has lasted more than 48 hours without concomitant anticoagulant therapy
- A TEE-guided cardioversion is equivalent to a standard approach of anticoagulation therapy 3 weeks before and 4 weeks after DCCV[22]

LONG-TERM MANAGEMENT OF AF IN PATIENTS WITH HF

A major treatment decision in the patient with HF with AF, is whether to pursue a rhythm control strategy over rate control for long-term management. Six major trials have been conducted to clarify the optimal treatment for AF (**Table 1**). Thus far, there is no compelling evidence that pharmacologic maintenance of SR leads to a better outcome as compared with rate control.[23–31]

However, it is noteworthy that quite a few limitations must be considered with these initial studies. A significant number of cross overs between strategy options, adverse effects of antiarrhythmic drugs, and general ineffectiveness of drugs used for rhythm control may have contributed to the lack of benefit seen with a rhythm-control strategy. In addition, therapy for stroke prophylaxis differed between treatment approaches and may have contributed to differences in outcome, biasing benefit toward the rate-control option.

Post hoc subgroup analyses from these large studies suggest a higher likelihood of survival in patients who were maintained in SR.[32–34] However, extrapolation of these data to the HF population is difficult because of the low number of patients with HF in the study sample. For example, in the Atrial Fibrillation Follow-up Investigation of Rhythm Management (AFFIRM) trial, only 23% of the study population had HF.[26] A more contemporary study by the Atrial Fibrillation and Congestive Heart Failure Investigators (AF-CHF trial), focused solely on a population with HF (n = 1376).[31] However, this study also failed to show superiority of rhythm control over rate control with respect to cardiovascular mortality.

Improvement in left ventricular ejection fraction (LVEF), n-terminal pro-brain natriuretic protein, and quality of life has also been reported in smaller studies with rhythm control strategies.[33] However, these results have yet to be replicated in larger trials. Despite the lack of mortality benefit from the rhythm-controlling strategy with antiarrhythmic drug therapy in AF-CHF, there was no increased cost associated with the strategy.[35]

IS RHYTHM CONTROL EVER THE RIGHT ANSWER?

Frequently patients with HF have substantial symptoms while in AF as compared to when they are in SR. Significant benefit may be achieved with return of the left atrial contribution to stroke volume in certain patients with HF. Thus, rhythm restoration is generally considered acceptable when patients with HF exhibit more than minimal symptoms. Conversely, rate control is the backbone of therapy if symptomatology does not differ significantly between SR and AF.

It should be noted, however, that a population of patients with systolic HF and atrial fibrillation

Table 1
Major trials comparing rate versus rhythm control strategy for atrial fibrillation

Trial, Year	Total No. of Patients	Patients with Heart Failure, %	Mean Age, y	Mean Follow-up, y	Rhythm Control Group	Rate Control Group	Outcomes
PIAF,[23,24] 2000	252	4	60.5	1	Amiodarone or DCCV	Diltiazem, BB, Digoxin or AVNA + PM	No significant differences in quality of life in patients in sinus rhythm or AF
AFFIRM,[26] 2002	4060	23	70	3.5	Amiodarone, sotalol, propafenone, procainamide	Digoxin, BB, Diltiazem, Verapamil	No significant differences in all-cause mortality; trend toward increased mortality with rhythm control
RACE,[28] 2002	522	50	68	2.3	Sotalol, flecainide, propafenone, amiodarone	Digoxin, CCB, BB	No significant differences in composite end point (cardiovascular death, CHF, embolic events, bleeding, pacemaker, severe adverse effects of AADs)
STAF,[29] 2003	200	56	65.8	1.6	Class I, sotalol, amiodarone	BB, Digoxin, CCB or AVNA + PM	No significant differences in composite end point (CPR, death, cerebrovascular and embolic events)
HOT CAFE,[30] 2004	205	46	60.8	1.7	Disopyramide, propafenone, sotalol, amiodarone	BB, CCB, Digoxin or AVNA + PM	No significant differences in composite end point (all-cause mortality, embolic events or major bleeding)
AF-CHF,[31] 2008	1376	100	66.5	3.1	Amiodarone, sotalol, dofetilide, or DCCV	BB, Digoxin or AVNA + PM	No significant differences in cardiovascular death

Abbreviations: AF, atrial fibrillation; AVNA, atrioventricular nodal ablation; BB, beta-blocker; CCB, calcium channel blocker; CHF, congestive heart failure; CPR, cardiopulmonary resuscitation; DCCV, direct current cardioversion; PM, pacemaker.
Data from Refs. [24,26,28-31]

(particularly rapid atrial fibrillation) may have developed HF directly as a result of atrial fibrillation.[36] When no other etiology is isolated, tachycardia-induced cardiomyopathy may be diagnosed. In this situation, rhythm control of atrial fibrillation is the preferred option with the goal of sustained rhythm control and resolution of the cardiomyopathy.[37]

MEDICAL THERAPY WITH RATE CONTROL: BETA-BLOCKERS, CALCIUM CHANNEL BLOCKERS, AND DIGOXIN

Beta-blockers, which also serve as evidenced-based treatment in systolic HF, are generally first-line for rate control via their effect on the AV node. As expected, a retrospective analysis of the US Carvedilol Heart Failure Trial established improved outcomes in patients with HF with concomitant AF who were in the treatment group.[38] Similar in their effect on the AV node, the *nondihydropyridine CCBs* (including verapamil and diltiazem) also are effective rate-controlling agents. As discussed previously, at optimal doses for ventricular rate control, CCBs are generally not tolerated in the low LVEF patients.[39]

Digoxin not only increases the refractory period, but also triggers vagal activation to slow the conduction of electrical impulses through the AV node. As mentioned previously, it is less effective in states of increased sympathetic tone, such as exercise or worsening HF.[2] However, digoxin does have a synergistic effect with beta-blockers as evidenced by the improvement in survival of patients' concomitantly on carvedilol and digoxin in a retrospective analysis of the US Carvedilol Heart Failure Trials.[38] Given the very narrow therapeutic window of digoxin, it is recommended that serum levels be maintained at less than 1.0 ng/mL.[40] In patients with HF with AF, digoxin may be considered as an adjuvant therapy.

HOW LOW TO GO?

The Lenient versus Strict Rate Control in Patients with Atrial Fibrillation study (RACE II) compared strict rate control (resting heart rate <80 beats per minute) versus lenient rate control (resting heart rate <110 beats per minute).[41] In a cohort of more than 600 patients with permanent atrial fibrillation, randomization to a lenient strategy was not inferior to a strict strategy in terms of cardiovascular mortality, malignant arrhythmias, and rate of hospitalizations during a 3-year follow-up.[41]

The RACE II study has noteworthy limitations when applying it to the HF population that must be appreciated. The population studied was relatively healthy, with only approximately 10% of patients having a history of HF hospitalization and only 15% with a known LVEF of 40% or less.[41] Nonetheless, even with limited data, lenient heart control is a practical initial approach. If symptoms continue despite more aggressive control of rate, then a rhythm-control strategy may be needed.

RHYTHM CONTROL

In the chronic setting, pharmacologic options for maintenance of SR in patients with HF are limited. Class I antiarrhythmics, sodium channel blockers, are contraindicated in HF, given their propensity to promote reentry in the structurally abnormal heart leading to VT.[42] The options for therapy in patients with HF and AF include dofetilide, amiodarone, and, to a lesser degree, sotalol and dronedarone (**Table 2**).

Dofetilide is a class III antiarrhythmic that induces potassium channel blockade (I_{Kr}). It is renally cleared and requires dosing based on creatinine clearance.[43] The Efficacy of Dofetilide in the Treatment of Atrial Fibrillation-Flutter in Patients with Reduced Left Ventricular Function (DIAMOND) substudy randomized 506 patients with AF or atrial flutter to either treatment with dofetilide or placebo.[34] Of note, this included a relatively high-risk population, with more than 50% having New York Heart Association (NYHA) class III or IV symptoms. Among 234 patients who achieved restoration of SR, patients were more likely to remain in SR at 1 year on dofetilide over placebo (79% vs 42%). Importantly, dofetilide's safety was proven in this cohort, with similar mortality between the treatment and placebo group. Interestingly, mortality was lower in patients who had SR restored and maintained, which was independent of therapy.[34] In general, dofetilide is considered more effective in the maintenance of SR than it is for cardioversion.[44]

Despite its efficacy, the use of dofetilide as an antiarrhythmic agent for AF in clinical practice has been limited.[45] This is largely due to the US Food and Drug Administration's (FDA's) mandatory requirement that initiation of this agent requires a minimum 72-hour in-hospital monitoring period. As a consequence of its potassium channel blocking effects, it carries a significant risk of torsades de pointes.[46] This effect is generally encountered within the first 3 days of initiation and thus close monitoring of the QT interval is necessary.[47]

Amiodarone is a unique antiarrhythmic with multiple channel effects. It inhibits adrenergic stimulation (with alpha-blocking and beta-blocking properties) and blocks sodium, potassium, and calcium channels. Despite not being FDA approved for AF,

Table 2
Membrane active antiarrhythmic drugs

Vaughn-Williams Classification	Medication	Channel/Receptor Action*				Mechanism of Action	Side Effects	Comments
		Na	K	Alpha	Beta			
Ia	Procainamide	↓	↓			• Slows conduction velocity • Increases refractoriness	• QT prolongation, TdP • Hypotension	• Monitor for hypotension • Contraindicated in impaired real function • Discontinue if QRS prolongation >50%
Ib	Lidocaine (intravenous) Mexiletine (oral)	↓				• Slows conduction velocity • Shortens refractoriness	• Drowsiness, visual disturbance, tinnitus • Seizure, obtundation (rare)	• Selectively acts on ischemic myocardium • Monitor concentration if using for >24 h
Ic	Flecainide	↓				• Slows conduction velocity	• Dizziness, headache, GI upset, blurred vision	• Contraindicated in CHD, significant LVH • Monitor for QT prolongation (first 3 d)
	Sotalol				↓	• Increases refractoriness • Blocks sympathetic activity • Decreases automaticity	• Dizziness, fatigue • QT prolongation, TdP • Bradycardia	• Dose-related TdP • Renally cleared

	Drug		Electrophysiologic effects	Adverse effects	Monitoring / Comments
III	Dofetilide	↓	• Increases refractoriness	• QT prolongation, TdP • Bradycardia	• Monitor for QT prolongation (first 3 d) • Dose-related TdP • Renally cleared • Contraindicated with verapamil, azoles, thiazide
	Azilimide				
	Amiodarone	↓ ↓ ↓ ↓	• Increases refractoriness • Long half-life • Slows conduction velocity • Increases refractoriness • Blocks sympathetic activity • Decreases automaticity	• QT prolongation, TdP • Toxicity: thyroid, pulmonary, liver, GI, skin, eyes • Bradycardia • <0.5% TdP	• Not available in the US • LFT, TFT every 6 mo • Ophthalmology annually • Monitor for symptoms: pulmonary, neurologic
	Dronedarone	↓ ↓	• Short half-life • Slows conduction velocity • Increases refractoriness • Blocks sympathetic activity • Decreases automaticity	• Toxicity: less than amiodarone	• Avoid in NYHA class III/IV, severe systolic dysfunction • Contraindicated in persistent AF

Abbreviations: AF, atrial fibrillation; CHD, coronary heart disease; GI, gastrointestinal; LFT, liver function test; LVH, left ventricular hypertrophy; NYHA, New York Heart Association; TdP, Torsades de pointes; TFT, thyroid function test.

* Downward arrow denotes site of primary cardiac channel blockade.

amiodarone is the most commonly prescribed drug for AF.[45] Amiodarone has long been considered by cardiologists to be the most effective antiarrhythmic for the suppression of AF. It should be noted there are no head-to-head trials comparing amiodarone with dofetilide. The Canadian Trail of Atrial Fibrillation (CTAF) and the Amiodarone versus Sotalol for Atrial Fibrillation (SAFE-T) trial both demonstrated superiority of amiodarone in maintenance of SR at follow-up in comparison with sotalol.[48,49] The use of amiodarone has been documented in patients with HF with LVEF of 40% or less to confer a greater likelihood of conversion to SR over placebo. Furthermore, patients that reverted to SR with amiodarone had a lower total mortality than those who did not.[32]

The primary cardiovascular side effect of amiodarone in patients with HF is symptomatic sinus bradycardia, with a higher predominance of females requiring permanent pacemaker insertion.[50,51] While QT prolongation can occur given its potassium channel blockade properties, amiodarone very rarely induces torsades de pointes at less than 0.5%.[52]

Unfortunately, amiodarone is fraught with many noncardiac toxicities that require careful surveillance.[53] Hepatotoxicity ranging from low-level transaminase elevation to full out fulminant liver failure can occur. The pulmonary toxicity induced by amiodarone can manifest in numerous ways. Adult respiratory distress syndromes, acute hypersensitivity reactions with patchy infiltrates, solitary pulmonary nodules, and a chronic interstitial fibrosis are all reported in the literature.[54] Both hypo- or hyperthyroidism may also occur with use. Hypothyroidism, generally induced by a destructive thyroiditis phenomena, is more common.[55]

Sotalol blocks the same potassium current as dofetilide and is also renally cleared. The racemic d,l-sotalol formulation, which is the only available formulation in the United States, is also a nonselective beta blocker.[56] The Survival With Oral d-Sotalol (SWORD) investigators found that in survivors of myocardial infarctions with depressed ejection fractions, the use of d-sotalol was associated with higher mortality from ventricular arrhythmias.[57] Expert opinion suggest the use of sotalol only for those systolic HF patients with cardiac defibrillators in place. As discussed previously, sotalol is inferior to amiodarone for maintenance of SR when compared head-to-head.[49]

Dronedarone is a newer drug that was designed to mimic the antiarrhythmic effects of amiodarone but with a milder side effect profile. It was initially promising in the general AF population, as it was shown to be more effective over placebo in maintaining SR, but without the lung and thyroid effects seen with amiodarone.[58] However, the 2007

ANDROMEDA trial, which examined the use of dronedarone in symptomatic patients with HF (NYHA class III/IV) with severe LV dysfunction (LVEF <35%) tempered enthusiasm for its use in patients with HF. The trial was halted early because of a significant increase in death in the dronedarone group at a median follow-up of 2 months.[59] Consequently, current recommendations by the FDA are that dronedarone be avoided in patients with HF with recent decompensation or in those with advanced disease (NYHA class III/IV or severe systolic dysfunction of the left ventricle).

NONPHARMACOLOGIC APPROACHES TO RHYTHM CONTROL

AV node ablation with biventricular pacemaker implantation has been shown in small trials to be effective in patients with HF with AF and rapid ventricular response that is refractory to medical therapy.[60] Manolis and colleagues[60] demonstrated a significant improvement in LVEF in a subgroup analysis of 30 patients with HF and atrial tachyarrhythmias who underwent an "ablate and pace" strategy. At 2-year follow-up, the LVEF improved from 32% ± 9% to 48% ± 8% and NYHA functional class also improved. A recent, larger systematic review of this approach was looked at in patients with HF with concomitant AF and cardiac resynchronization therapy. Ganesan and colleagues[61] pooled mortality data from 450 patients across 3 nonrandomized trials and showed that AV node ablation in patients with HF with AF was associated with a reduction in all-cause and cardiovascular mortality. Prospective, randomized controlled trials are needed to confirm these results.

AV nodal ablation with biventricular pacing was compared with pulmonary vein isolation (PVI) for benefit of HF status in 81 patients with drug-refractory AF and LVEF of 40% or less.[62] It was found that PVI was superior to AV node ablation with biventricular pacing in improvement of LVEF and quality of life assessed by the Minnesota Living with Heart Failure questionnaire. At 6 months, the LVEF had improved in the PVI group from 28% up to 35% (P<.001).[62]

Catheter ablation of atrial fibrillation is quickly becoming a promising new therapeutic intervention in symptomatic patients with HF when rate-control and antiarrhythmic drugs have failed. Radiofrequency ablation performs superiorly to antiarrhythmic drug therapy in the maintenance of SR.[63] Tondo and colleagues[64] reported a success rate of 88% for maintaining SR at 1 year in patients undergoing PVI with impaired LV function.

Catheter-based ablation strategies also appear to improve LVEF and quality of life while increasing exertional tolerance in nonrandomized trials. The ARC-HF trial examined 52 symptomatic patients with HF with LVEF of 35% or less and randomly assigned them to a rate control strategy versus PVI. At 12 months, peak oxygen consumption and quality-of-life scores were appreciably improved.[65] Hsu and colleagues[66] found improvement in LV chamber size and mean LVEF from 35% to 56% in 58 patients with HF who underwent PVI.

The data for nonpharmacologic treatment of AF in HF continues to grow. The efficacy and safety of catheter-based procedures is also steadily improving.[67] However, the benefit of catheter ablation must be balanced with the procedural risk in patients with HF. Sufficient data are currently lacking to make strong recommendations regarding where in the therapeutic approach catheter ablation of AF should fall in patients with HF. The 2013 American College of Cardiology Foundation/American Heart Association HF guidelines give a IIB recommendation for ablation in patients with HF with persistent AF and the presence of disabling symptoms when antiarrhythmic therapy has failed.[39]

VENTRICULAR ARRHYTHMIAS IN HF

Sudden cardiac death (SCD) is a sudden, unexpected death caused by loss of heart function. Half of all the heart disease deaths, or more than 350,000 deaths annually, in the United States are due to SCD.[68,69] Life-threatening ventricular arrhythmias, including VT and ventricular fibrillation (VF) are responsible for most sudden deaths.[70] Ventricular arrhythmias occur with a much higher prevalence in those with HF with reduced ejection fraction (HFrEF). In fact, the primary mode of death in patients with NYHA I, II, or III HF is sudden death due to ventricular arrhythmia.[71]

MECHANISMS FOR VENTRICULAR ARRHYTHMIA AND ANTIARRHYTHMIC DRUG THERAPY IN HF

Multiple potential factors contribute to the development of ventricular arrhythmias in patients with HF (Fig. 2)[72,73]:

- Myocardial fibrosis leads to loss of cell-cell coupling, resulting in slowed electrical conduction and providing a substrate for reentry
- Abnormal triggered activity provides a focal mechanism for arrhythmia
- Repolarization of myocardial cells is altered due to disruption of outward potassium current
- Ventricular dilatation contributes to alterations in action potential refractoriness and conduction

- Sympathetic activation promotes abnormal automaticity and precipitates triggered activity
- Activation of the angiotensin system leads to electrolyte disturbance, promoting arrhythmia
- Subendocardial ischemia manifests as enhanced automaticity and regional alteration in conduction velocity and refractoriness, which are proarrhythmic
- Drugs commonly used in the treatment of HF, including inotropes, phosphodiesterase inhibitors, and digoxin can be proarrhythmic

Antiarrhythmic drugs have mechanistic effects, which counter those contributing to the genesis of ventricular arrhythmias (see Table 2). Drugs used for the treatment of ventricular arrhythmia include the following:

- Class Ia antiarrhythmics (eg, procainamide) slow conduction velocity and increase refractoriness
- Class Ib antiarrhythmics (eg, lidocaine, mexiletine) slow conduction velocity and shorten refractoriness, particularly in ischemic myocardium
- Class II antiarrhythmics (beta-blockers) block sympathetic activity and reduce conduction velocity
- Class III antiarrhythmics (sotalol, dofetilide, azimilide) increase refractoriness
- Amiodarone or dronedarone are drugs with combined effects that slow conduction velocity, block sympathetic activity, and increase refractoriness

The use of ICDs has revolutionized the care of the patient with HF. However, ICDs only provide a rescue therapy for ventricular arrhythmia and do not prevent the occurrence of arrhythmia. It has been well established that patients with HF with an ICD for primary prevention have a higher mortality risk if they receive a shock.[74] Furthermore, the anxiety and anguish that some patients experience from repeated shocks can be debilitating.[75] The fact that ICD shocks portend a poor prognosis in patients with HF,[74] and have profound psychological consequences, emphasizes the need to prevent and treat ventricular arrhythmias. In this role, antiarrhythmic drug therapy plays a pivotal role.

ANTIARRHYTHMIC DRUG THERAPY FOR PRIMARY PROPHYLAXIS OF VENTRICULAR ARRHYTHMIA IN PATIENTS WITH HF

Ventricular arrhythmias claim a significant number of lives of patients with HFrEF. Thus, many of the antiarrhythmic drugs (AAD) have been studied for

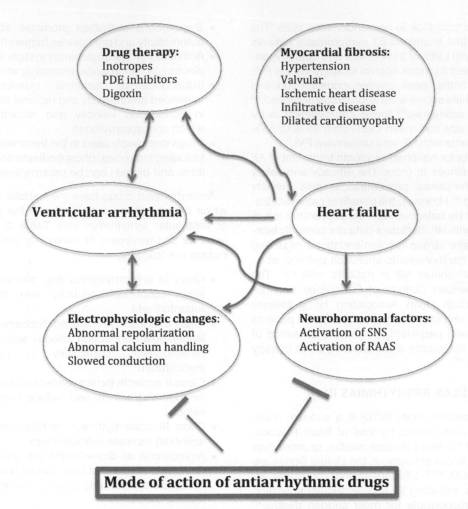

Fig. 2. HF induces neurohormonal activation, structural remodeling, and electrophysiologic changes, all of which can stimulate ventricular arrhythmias. Furthermore, certain drug therapy used in HF can also contribute to a proarrhythmic state. PDE, phosphodiesterase inhibitors; RAAS, renin-angiotensin-aldosterone system; SNS, sympathetic nervous system.

the primary prophylaxis of ventricular arrhythmias, including the following:

Beta-blockers

- Metoprolol (MERIT-HF) and Bisoprolol (CIBIS-II), both lipophilic and highly β1 selective beta-blockers, have been shown to reduce the risk for sudden cardiac death by 41% and 44%, respectively.[71,76]
- Carvedilol is a nonselective β1, β2, and α blocker. The US Carvedilol Heart Failure Study group[77] showed the benefit of carvedilol in reducing the risk of VT/VF in patients with HF.

Sotalol

- Sotalol was studied in the SWORD trial.[60] The d-sotalol was compared with placebo in 3121

patients with LVEF of 40% or less and recent (6–42 days) myocardial infarction (MI) or symptomatic congestive heart failure (CHF) in the setting of a remote (≥42 days) MI. The trial was terminated prematurely because all-cause mortality (5.0% vs 3.1%) and arrhythmic death (3.6% vs 2.0%) were significantly higher with sotalol as compared with placebo.

Amiodarone

- In the EMIAT trial, amiodarone in comparison with placebo resulted in a 35% reduction in arrhythmic death ($P = .05$) in survivors of myocardial infarction with an EF 40% or less; however, there was no significant difference in all-cause or cardiac mortality.[78,79]

- The Grupo de Estudio de la Sobrevida en la Insuficiencia Cardiaca en Argentina (GESICA) study showed a nonsignificant risk reduction (27%; P = .16) of sudden death with amiodarone as compared with placebo in severe HF.[80]
- Amiodarone did not reduce mortality compared with placebo in the Sudden Cardiac Death in Heart Failure Trial (SCD-HeFT),[81] which looked at patients with an LVEF of 35% or less and NYHA II or III HF.
- A meta-analysis of 15 randomized controlled trials examining the use of amiodarone versus placebo/control for the prevention of SCD in 8522 patients showed that there was a 1.5% absolute risk reduction in all-cause mortality that was not statistically significant (P = .093).[82]

Dronedarone

- The Antiarrhythmic Trial with Dronedarone in Moderate-to-Severe Congestive Heart Failure Evaluating Morbidity Decrease (ANDROMEDA)[59] evaluated patients with NYHA class III or IV symptoms and EF of 35% or less. The trial was terminated early due to a significantly higher mortality rate with dronedarone treatment (8.1%) as compared with placebo (3.8%).

Dofetilide

- The DIAMOND-MI trial enrolled 1510 patients within 2 to 7 days of an acute MI with an EF of 35% or less. Patients were randomly assigned to receive either dofetilide (n = 749) or placebo (n = 761).[83] There was no difference in arrhythmic death or mortality.
- The DIAMOND-CHF trial consisted of patients with LVEF of 35% or less who were hospitalized for new or worsening CHF within 7 days.[47] Dofetilide use did not result in a significant difference in SCD or mortality.

Azimilide

- Azimilide is a newer class III AAD that is currently available only in Europe.
- Azimilide Post-Infarct Survival Evaluation (ALIVE)[84] trial looked at 3717 patients after an MI with an EF between 15% and 35% who were randomized to azimilide or placebo. No significant difference was found in arrhythmic deaths or mortality.

Several studies have shown that *beta-blockers* remain among the very few AADs that reduce the incidence of SCD and prolong survival. Once patients are treated with evidence-based therapies for HF, evidence suggests that there is no role for other antiarrhythmic drug therapy in the primary prevention of ventricular arrhythmias.

ACUTE MANAGEMENT OF UNSTABLE VENTRICULAR ARRHYTHMIA IN PATIENTS WITH HF

Management of acute ventricular arrhythmia in patients with HF is challenging and requires an approach tailored to the underlying cause. Acute management of the hemodynamically unstable patient is according to the algorithm outlined by Advanced Cardiovascular Life Support (ACLS) guidelines, including cardiopulmonary resuscitation, defibrillation, a vasoactive agent (epinephrine or vasopressin), and/or amiodarone. Following acute resuscitation, the management should shift to determining and correcting the underlying instigator. This may range from volume overload/acute on chronic decompensation, ischemia, electrolyte imbalances, or other causative factors.

MANAGEMENT OF STABLE VENTRICULAR ARRHYTHMIA IN PATIENTS WITH HF

In the hemodynamically stable patient with VT, acute management may include sedation with synchronized cardioversion or infusion of procainamide, lidocaine, or amiodarone.

Before treatment, careful consideration must be given to distinguishing the presenting rhythm as VT versus SVT with aberrant conduction or much more rarely a preexcited tachycardia. This should be done by careful examination of the 12-lead electrocardiogram during tachycardia in combination with the clinical context. In the patients with HF, because VT is more prevalent, this should be the presumed diagnosis unless proven otherwise.

Once the diagnosis of VT is made, efforts should be made to terminate the VT. Sedation with cardioversion can be considered a primary option. However, antiarrhythmic agents are often used.

Procainamide is a class la antiarrhythmic agent that blocks fast sodium channels in addition to being a potent potassium channel blocker. The parent compound primarily blocks sodium channels, whereas its metabolite, N-acetylprocainamide, blocks potassium channels. The potassium channel blocking effect of N-acetylprocainamide is likely the primary mode for its high rate of VT termination.[85,86] Because of its potassium channel blocking effect, procainamide can be proarrhythmic (torsade de pointes), particularly in those with impaired renal function. Procainamide is typically given as a slow load of 10 to 15 mg/kg or until VT terminates, followed by an infusion of 1 to 4 mg per minute. Due to its alpha-blocking properties, procainamide can cause hypotension.[87] Procainamide should be used cautiously in the patient with HF.

Lidocaine is a class Ib antiarrhythmic agent, which preferentially blocks inactivated sodium channels. Conditions that enhance the utility of lidocaine are more prevalent with ischemic VT. In other situations, lidocaine may not be as effective as procainamide.[86] Lidocaine is given as a load of 1.0 to 1.5 mg/kg that can be repeated at a dose of 0.5 to 0.75 mg/kg followed by a continuous infusion of 1 to 4 mg/min. The primary side effects to watch for are neurologic (visual disturbances, confusion, drowsiness, seizures).

Although amiodarone is frequently used in the acute treatment of stable VT, it is not ideal for acute cardioversion. Amiodarone blocks fast sodium channels in a fashion similar to lidocaine, in addition to having beta-blocker and calcium-channel blocker properties. However, its effect on ventricular refractoriness may take weeks to develop.[88,89] Thus, amiodarone is more effective as a long-term agent to prevent recurrent arrhythmia. Fortunately, amiodarone has minimal negative inotropic effects and rarely is proarrhythmic.

Recurrent ventricular arrhythmia, including electrical storm, defined as 3 or more events in 24 hours, may require further therapy including multiple antiarrhythmic agents, nonpharmacologic treatment, such as rapid pacing, radiofrequency ablation, deep sedation, and in extreme circumstances, temporary mechanical circulatory support or heart transplantation.

Beta-blocker therapy is an important adjunctive therapy to any membrane-active antiarrhythmic in both the acute and chronic management of ventricular arrhythmia. Clearly, as discussed previously, there are beneficial effects of beta-blocker therapy in preventing recurrent ventricular arrhythmia. Furthermore, beta-blocker therapy is a fundamental component of medical therapy in patients with HF. However, beta-blocker therapy is also beneficial in acute management of ventricular arrhythmia. Blocking sympathetic activity with a beta-blocker or stellate ganglion blockade not only decreases the propensity for ventricular arrhythmia but also increases the VF threshold.[90]

ANTIARRHYTHMIC DRUGS FOR SECONDARY PREVENTION OF ICD SHOCKS

The use of ICDs in patients with HF has revolutionized their care and successfully extended the length of high-quality, high-functioning life for our patients with HF. However, although ICDs prevent sudden death, many patients will suffer ICD shocks, some with a relatively high frequency. Thus, we have moved from an era of ICD implantation to an era of shock reduction.

Shock reduction strategies encompass several approaches, including the following:

- Aggressive use of antitachycardia pacing (ATP)
- Device programming to withhold unnecessary shocks from SVT or nonsustained ventricular arrhythmias
- Drug-based or catheter-based therapy to prevent the occurrence of ventricular arrhythmias

In this role, antiarrhythmic drug therapy has a pivotal role in the secondary prevention of ICD shocks in patients with HF.

As described previously, *beta-blockers* should be a cornerstone of management for patients with HF. They are also effective in the reduction of ICD shocks. In a substudy of the Multicenter Automatic Defibrillator Implantation Trial (MADIT-II) evaluating the benefit of ICDs in primary prevention of SCD, patients who received beta-blockers had a 52% reduction in ventricular arrhythmic requiring ICD shock.[91]

Sotalol was studied for the prevention of ICD shock in a double-blind, prospective, multicenter trial by Pacifico and colleagues.[92] In this study, 302 patients were randomized to receive racemic d,l-sotalol or placebo and were followed for 12 months. Sotalol was associated with a 48% reduction in risk of mortality or first shock. This included a reduction in both inappropriate and appropriate shock. Those on sotalol were more likely to be bradycardic and have QT prolongation but there was only 1 case of torsade de point.[92]

Azimilide is a novel class III antiarrhythmic drug, currently available only in Europe. Azimilide blocks both the rapid and slow delayed rectifier potassium currents, unlike other class III antiarrhythmics (which block only the rapid rectifier potassium current). Azimilide has been shown to be effective in reducing ICD shocks in multiple studies. A pilot study of 172 patients by Singer and colleagues[93] demonstrated a 69% reduction in the relative risk of appropriate ICD shocks or antitachycardia pacing at 1 year. The larger Shock Inhibition Evaluation with Azimilide (SHIELD) study randomized 633 ICD patients to placebo, azimilide 75 mg, or azimilide 125 mg. At 1-year follow-up, the primary end point of all-cause ICD shock or ATP was reduced by 57% for the 75-mg dose and 47% for the 125-mg dose. The secondary end point of appropriate ICD shock or ATP was reduced by 48% for the 75-mg dose and 62% for the 125-mg dose. Adverse events with azimilide were low, including QT prolongation with torsade de point in 5 patients and reversible neutropenia in 1 patient. Further investigation with azimilide is awaited.[93]

Amiodarone remains the most efficacious and safe of the antiarrhythmic drugs for ICD shock prevention. The Optimal Pharmacologic Therapy in Cardioverter Defibrillator Patients (OPTIC) study compared the efficacy of beta-blocker alone, sotalol, or beta-blocker with amiodarone for the prevention of ICD shocks.[94] In this randomized controlled trial of 412 patients, at 1-year follow-up, amiodarone with beta-blocker reduced the risk of appropriate or inappropriate ICD shock by 73% compared with beta-blocker alone and by 57% compared with sotalol. However, adverse pulmonary, thyroid, and bradycardic events were more common with amiodarone compared with other therapies.[94]

OTHER EFFECTS OF ANTIARRHYTHMIC DRUG THERAPY IN ICD PATIENTS

Importantly, the use of antiarrhythmic drug therapy can have an effect on defibrillation and pacing thresholds. In general, class I agents (procainamide, lidocaine, mexiletine) and amiodarone can increase defibrillation and pacing threshold. On the other hand, class III agents (sotalol, dofetilide) can lower thresholds. In a substudy of the OPTIC trial, amiodarone led to a small 1.29-J increase in defibrillation threshold, whereas sotalol was associated with a 0.89-J reduction in defibrillation threshold and beta-blocker was associated with a 1.67-J reduction in threshold. In patients with a high defibrillation threshold and a low safety margin with ICD output, defibrillation threshold testing may be required in certain circumstances.[95]

It should also be noted that antiarrhythmic drugs can prolong the cycle length of ventricular arrhythmias. This can be problematic, as detection algorithms may need to be adjusted so that slow VT is appropriately detected after antiarrhythmic drug loading. Additionally, slow ventricular rhythms may become more resistant to therapy, as the excitable gap of the arrhythmia circuit widens.

SUMMARY

Structural remodeling, underlying neurohormonal activation, and concomitant drug therapies in patients with HF all create an ideal substrate for both atrial and ventricular arrhythmias. Although they commonly coexist, the presence of AF or VT in the HF patient adversely affects mortality. Beta-blockers remain the ideal treatment for rate control in the patient with AF and for both prevention and suppression of VT. Although antiarrhythmics can be proarrhythmic and have significant toxicities, when used cautiously, they can have an important role in the treatment of the patient with chronic HF. In patients with HF who remain persistently symptomatic despite adequate rate control, certain antiarrhythmics can be helpful for restoration of SR. Furthermore, their utility in the acute termination of ventricular arrhythmias and in the secondary prevention of ICD shocks has been well established.

REFERENCES

1. Blomström-Lundqvist C, Scheinman MM, Aliot EM, et al. ACC/AHA/ESC guidelines for the management of patients with supraventricular arrhythmias–executive summary. A report of the American College of Cardiology/American Heart Association Task Force on practice guidelines and the European Society of Cardiology. J Am Coll Cardiol 2003;42(8):1493–531. Available at: http://www.ncbi.nlm.nih.gov/pubmed/14563598. Accessed April 9, 2014.

2. Fuster V, Rydén LE, Cannom DS, et al. ACC/AHA/ESC 2006 guidelines for the management of patients with atrial fibrillation: a report of the American College of Cardiology/American Heart Association Task Force on practice guidelines and the European Society of Cardiology Committee for practice. Circulation 2006;114(7):e257–354. http://dx.doi.org/10.1161/CIRCULATIONAHA.106.177292.

3. Miyasaka Y, Barnes ME, Gersh BJ, et al. Secular trends in incidence of atrial fibrillation in Olmsted County, Minnesota, 1980 to 2000, and implications on the projections for future prevalence. Circulation 2006;114(2):119–25. http://dx.doi.org/10.1161/CIRCULATIONAHA.105.595140.

4. Jessup M, Brozena S. Heart failure. N Engl J Med 2003;348(20):2007–18. http://dx.doi.org/10.1056/NEJMra021498.

5. Roger VL, Go AS, Lloyd-Jones DM, et al. Heart disease and stroke statistics–2011 update: a report from the American Heart Association. Circulation 2011;123(4):e18–209. http://dx.doi.org/10.1161/CIR.0b013e3182009701.

6. Verheule S, Wilson E, Everett T, et al. Alterations in atrial electrophysiology and tissue structure in a canine model of chronic atrial dilatation due to mitral regurgitation. Circulation 2003;107(20):2615–22. http://dx.doi.org/10.1161/01.CIR.0000066915.15187.51.

7. De Mello WC. Cell coupling and impulse propagation in the failing heart. J Cardiovasc Electrophysiol 1999;10(10):1409–20. Available at: http://www.ncbi.nlm.nih.gov/pubmed/10515566. Accessed April 21, 2014.

8. Tomaselli GF, Rose J. Molecular aspects of arrhythmias associated with cardiomyopathies. Curr Opin Cardiol 2000;15(3):202–8. Available at: http://www.ncbi.nlm.nih.gov/pubmed/10952429. Accessed April 21, 2014.

9. Cooper HA, Dries DL, Davis CE, et al. Diuretics and risk of arrhythmic death in patients with left ventricular dysfunction. Circulation 1999;100(12):1311–5. Available at: http://www.ncbi.nlm.nih.gov/pubmed/10491376. Accessed April 21, 2014.

10. Gage BF, Waterman AD, Shannon W, et al. Validation of clinical classification schemes for predicting stroke: results from the National Registry of Atrial Fibrillation. JAMA 2001;285(22):2864–70. Available at: http://www.ncbi.nlm.nih.gov/pubmed/11401607. Accessed March 20, 2014.

11. Stevenson WG, Stevenson LW, Middlekauff HR, et al. Improving survival for patients with atrial fibrillation and advanced heart failure. J Am Coll Cardiol 1996; 28(6):1458–63. Available at: http://www.ncbi.nlm.nih.gov/pubmed/8917258. Accessed April 7, 2014.

12. Linssen GC, Rienstra M, Jaarsma T, et al. Clinical and prognostic effects of atrial fibrillation in heart failure patients with reduced and preserved left ventricular ejection fraction. Eur J Heart Fail 2011;13(10):1111–20. http://dx.doi.org/10.1093/eurjhf/hfr066.

13. Neuberger H-R, Mewis C, van Veldhuisen DJ, et al. Management of atrial fibrillation in patients with heart failure. Eur Heart J 2007;28(21):2568–77. http://dx.doi.org/10.1093/eurheartj/ehm341.

14. Middlekauff HR, Stevenson WG, Stevenson LW. Prognostic significance of atrial fibrillation in advanced heart failure. A study of 390 patients. Circulation 1991;84(1):40–8. Available at: http://www.ncbi.nlm.nih.gov/pubmed/2060110. Accessed April 21, 2014.

15. Mamas MA, Caldwell JC, Chacko S, et al. A meta-analysis of the prognostic significance of atrial fibrillation in chronic heart failure. Eur J Heart Fail 2009;11(7):676–83. http://dx.doi.org/10.1093/eurjhf/hfp085.

16. Mahoney P, Kimmel S, DeNofrio D, et al. Prognostic significance of atrial fibrillation in patients at a tertiary medical center referred for heart transplantation because of severe heart failure. Am J Cardiol 1999;83(11):1544–7. Available at: http://www.ncbi.nlm.nih.gov/pubmed/10363868. Accessed March 27, 2014.

17. Crijns HJ, Tjeerdsma G, de Kam PJ, et al. Prognostic value of the presence and development of atrial fibrillation in patients with advanced chronic heart failure. Eur Heart J 2000;21(15):1238–45. http://dx.doi.org/10.1053/euhj.1999.2107.

18. Senni M, Tribouilloy CM, Rodeheffer RJ, et al. Congestive heart failure in the community: trends in incidence and survival in a 10-year period. Arch Intern Med 1999;159(1):29–34. Available at: http://www.ncbi.nlm.nih.gov/pubmed/9892327. Accessed April 21, 2014.

19. Heist EK, Mansour M, Ruskin JN. Rate control in atrial fibrillation: targets, methods, resynchronization considerations. Circulation 2011;124(24):2746–55. http://dx.doi.org/10.1161/CIRCULATIONAHA.111.019919.

20. Olshansky B, Rosenfeld LE, Warner AL, et al. The Atrial Fibrillation Follow-up Investigation of Rhythm Management (AFFIRM) study: approaches to control rate in atrial fibrillation. J Am Coll Cardiol 2004;43(7):1201–8. http://dx.doi.org/10.1016/j.jacc.2003.11.032.

21. Pagel PS, Hettrick DA, Kersten JR, et al. Cardiovascular effects of propofol in dogs with dilated cardiomyopathy. Anesthesiology 1998;88(1):180–9. Available at: http://www.ncbi.nlm.nih.gov/pubmed/9447871. Accessed April 21, 2014.

22. Klein AL, Grimm RA, Murray RD, et al. Use of transesophageal echocardiography to guide cardioversion in patients with atrial fibrillation. N Engl J Med 2001;344(19):1411–20. http://dx.doi.org/10.1056/NEJM200105103441901.

23. Hohnloser SH, Kuck KH, Lilienthal J. Rhythm or rate control in atrial fibrillation–Pharmacological Intervention in Atrial Fibrillation (PIAF): a randomised trial. Lancet 2000;356(9244):1789–94. Available at: http://www.ncbi.nlm.nih.gov/pubmed/11117910. Accessed April 21, 2014.

24. Hohnloser SH, Kuck KH. Randomized trial of rhythm or rate control in atrial fibrillation: the Pharmacological Intervention in Atrial Fibrillation Trial (PIAF). Eur Heart J 2001;22(10):801–2. http://dx.doi.org/10.1053/euhj.2001.2596.

25. Grönefeld GC, Lilienthal J, Kuck KH, et al. Impact of rate versus rhythm control on quality of life in patients with persistent atrial fibrillation. Results from a prospective randomized study. Eur Heart J 2003;24(15):1430–6. Available at: http://www.ncbi.nlm.nih.gov/pubmed/12909072. Accessed April 21, 2014.

26. Wyse DG, Waldo AL, DiMarco JP, et al. A comparison of rate control and rhythm control in patients with atrial fibrillation. N Engl J Med 2002;347(23):1825–33. http://dx.doi.org/10.1056/NEJMoa021328.

27. Steinberg JS, Sadaniantz A, Kron J, et al. Analysis of cause-specific mortality in the Atrial Fibrillation Follow-up Investigation of Rhythm Management (AFFIRM) study. Circulation 2004;109(16):1973–80. http://dx.doi.org/10.1161/01.CIR.0000118472.77237.FA.

28. Van Gelder IC, Hagens VE, Bosker HA, et al. A comparison of rate control and rhythm control in patients with recurrent persistent atrial fibrillation. N Engl J Med 2002;347(23):1834–40. http://dx.doi.org/10.1056/NEJMoa021375.

29. Carlsson J, Miketic S, Windeler J, et al. Randomized trial of rate-control versus rhythm-control in persistent atrial fibrillation: the Strategies of Treatment of Atrial Fibrillation (STAF) study. J Am Coll Cardiol 2003;41(10):1690–6. Available at: http://www.ncbi.nlm.nih.gov/pubmed/12767648. Accessed April 21, 2014.

30. Opolski G, Torbicki A, Kosior DA, et al. Rate control vs rhythm control in patients with nonvalvular persistent atrial fibrillation: the results of the Polish How to Treat Chronic Atrial Fibrillation (HOT CAFE) study. Chest 2004;126(2):476–86. http://dx.doi.org/10.1378/chest.126.2.476.

31. Roy D, Talajic M, Nattel S, et al. Rhythm control versus rate control for atrial fibrillation and heart failure. N Engl J Med 2008;358(25):2667–77. http://dx.doi.org/10.1056/NEJMoa0708789.

32. Deedwania PC, Singh BN, Ellenbogen K, et al. Spontaneous conversion and maintenance of sinus rhythm by amiodarone in patients with heart failure and atrial fibrillation: observations from the Veterans Affairs Congestive Heart Failure Survival Trial of Antiarrhythmic Therapy (CHF-STAT). The Department of Veterans Affairs CHF-STAT Investigators. Circulation 1998;98(23):2574–9. Available at: http://www.ncbi.nlm.nih.gov/pubmed/9843465. Accessed April 21, 2014.

33. Shelton RJ, Clark AL, Goode K, et al. A randomised, controlled study of rate versus rhythm control in patients with chronic atrial fibrillation and heart failure: (CAFE-II Study). Heart 2009; 95(11):924–30. http://dx.doi.org/10.1136/hrt.2008.158931.

34. Pedersen OD, Bagger H, Keller N, et al. Efficacy of dofetilide in the treatment of atrial fibrillation-flutter in patients with reduced left ventricular function: a Danish investigations of arrhythmia and mortality on dofetilide (diamond) substudy. Circulation 2001;104(3):292–6. Available at: http://www.ncbi.nlm.nih.gov/pubmed/11457747. Accessed April 21, 2014.

35. Poulin F, Khairy P, Roy D, et al. Atrial fibrillation and congestive heart failure: a cost analysis of rhythm-control vs. rate-control strategies. Can J Cardiol 2013;29(10):1256–62. http://dx.doi.org/10.1016/j.cjca.2013.03.005.

36. Whipple G, Sheffield L, Woodman E, et al. Reversible congestive heart failure due to rapid stimulation of the normal heart. In: Proc New Engl Cardiovasc Soc. 1961–1962;20:39–40.

37. Thihalolipavan S, Morin DP. Atrial fibrillation and congestive heart failure. Heart Fail Clin 2014; 10(2):305–18. http://dx.doi.org/10.1016/j.hfc.2013.12.005.

38. Joglar JA, Acusta AP, Shusterman NH, et al. Effect of carvedilol on survival and hemodynamics in patients with atrial fibrillation and left ventricular dysfunction: retrospective analysis of the US Carvedilol Heart Failure Trials Program. Am Heart J 2001;142(3):498–501. http://dx.doi.org/10.1067/mhj.2001.117318.

39. Yancy CW, Jessup M, Bozkurt B, et al. 2013 ACCF/AHA guideline for the management of heart failure: a report of the American College of Cardiology Foundation/American Heart Association Task Force on practice guidelines. J Am Coll Cardiol 2013; 62(16):e147–239. http://dx.doi.org/10.1016/j.jacc.2013.05.019.

40. Rathore SS, Curtis JP, Wang Y, et al. Association of serum digoxin concentration and outcomes in patients with heart failure. JAMA 2003;289(7):871–8. Available at: http://www.ncbi.nlm.nih.gov/pubmed/12588271. Accessed April 23, 2014.

41. Van Gelder IC, Groenveld HF, Crijns HJ, et al. Lenient versus strict rate control in patients with atrial fibrillation. N Engl J Med 2010;362(15):1363–73. http://dx.doi.org/10.1056/NEJMoa1001337.

42. Zimetbaum P. Antiarrhythmic drug therapy for atrial fibrillation. Circulation 2012;125(2):381–9. http://dx.doi.org/10.1161/CIRCULATIONAHA.111.019927.

43. Walker DK, Alabaster CT, Congrave GS, et al. Significance of metabolism in the disposition and action of the antidysrhythmic drug, dofetilide. In vitro studies and correlation with in vivo data. Drug Metab Dispos 1996;24(4):447–55. Available at: http://www.ncbi.nlm.nih.gov/pubmed/8801060. Accessed April 23, 2014.

44. Singh S, Zoble RG, Yellen L, et al. Efficacy and safety of oral dofetilide in converting to and maintaining sinus rhythm in patients with chronic atrial fibrillation or atrial flutter: the symptomatic atrial fibrillation investigative research on dofetilide (SAFIRE-D) study. Circulation 2000;102(19):2385–90. Available at: http://www.ncbi.nlm.nih.gov/pubmed/11067793. Accessed April 23, 2014.

45. IMS Health. National Prescription Audit(TM): 1998 - 2006; Plymouth Meeting; PA. IMS Health; 2010. (Extracted Jan 2011).

46. Mazur A, Anderson ME, Bonney S, et al. Pause-dependent polymorphic ventricular tachycardia during long-term treatment with dofetilide: a placebo-controlled, implantable cardioverter-defibrillator-based evaluation. J Am Coll Cardiol 2001;37(4):1100–5. Available at: http://www.ncbi.nlm.nih.gov/pubmed/11263615. Accessed April 23, 2014.

47. Torp-Pedersen C, Møller M, Bloch-Thomsen PE, et al. Dofetilide in patients with congestive heart failure and left ventricular dysfunction. Danish Investigations of Arrhythmia and Mortality on Dofetilide Study Group. N Engl J Med 1999;341(12):857–65. http://dx.doi.org/10.1056/NEJM199909163411201.

48. Singh BN, Singh SN, Reda DJ, et al. Amiodarone versus sotalol for atrial fibrillation. N Engl J Med

2005;352(18):1861–72. http://dx.doi.org/10.1056/NEJMoa041705.

49. Roy D, Talajic M, Dorian P, et al. Amiodarone to prevent recurrence of atrial fibrillation. Canadian Trial of Atrial Fibrillation Investigators. N Engl J Med 2000;342(13):913–20. http://dx.doi.org/10.1056/NEJM200003303421302.

50. Essebag V, Reynolds MR, Hadjis T, et al. Sex differences in the relationship between amiodarone use and the need for permanent pacing in patients with atrial fibrillation. Arch Intern Med 2007;167(15):1648–53. http://dx.doi.org/10.1001/archinte.167.15.1648.

51. Weinfeld MS, Drazner MH, Stevenson WG, et al. Early outcome of initiating amiodarone for atrial fibrillation in advanced heart failure. J Heart Lung Transplant 2000;19(7):638–43. Available at: http://www.ncbi.nlm.nih.gov/pubmed/10930812. Accessed April 23, 2014.

52. Kaufman ES, Zimmermann PA, Wang T, et al. Risk of proarrhythmic events in the Atrial Fibrillation Follow-up Investigation of Rhythm Management (AFFIRM) study: a multivariate analysis. J Am Coll Cardiol 2004;44(6):1276–82. http://dx.doi.org/10.1016/j.jacc.2004.06.052.

53. Zimetbaum P. Amiodarone for atrial fibrillation. N Engl J Med 2007;356(9):935–41. http://dx.doi.org/10.1056/NEJMct065916.

54. Dusman RE, Stanton MS, Miles WM, et al. Clinical features of amiodarone-induced pulmonary toxicity. Circulation 1990;82(1):51–9. Available at: http://www.ncbi.nlm.nih.gov/pubmed/2364524. Accessed April 23, 2014.

55. Cohen-Lehman J, Dahl P, Danzi S, et al. Effects of amiodarone therapy on thyroid function. Nat Rev Endocrinol 2010;6(1):34–41. http://dx.doi.org/10.1038/nrendo.2009.225.

56. Ellison KE, Stevenson WG, Sweeney MO, et al. Management of arrhythmias in heart failure. Congest Heart Fail 2003;9(2):91–9. Available at: http://www.ncbi.nlm.nih.gov/pubmed/12671340. Accessed April 23, 2014.

57. Waldo AL, Camm AJ, DeRuyter H, et al. Effect of d-sotalol on mortality in patients with left ventricular dysfunction after recent and remote myocardial infarction. The SWORD Investigators. Survival With Oral d-Sotalol. Lancet 1996;348(9019):7–12. Available at: http://www.ncbi.nlm.nih.gov/pubmed/8691967. Accessed April 23, 2014.

58. Singh BN, Connolly SJ, Crijns HJ, et al. Dronedarone for maintenance of sinus rhythm in atrial fibrillation or flutter. N Engl J Med 2007;357(10):987–99. http://dx.doi.org/10.1056/NEJMoa054686.

59. Køber L, Torp-Pedersen C, McMurray JJ, et al. Increased mortality after dronedarone therapy for severe heart failure. N Engl J Med 2008;358(25):2678–87. http://dx.doi.org/10.1056/NEJMoa0800456.

60. Manolis AG, Katsivas AG, Lazaris EE, et al. Ventricular performance and quality of life in patients who underwent radiofrequency AV junction ablation and permanent pacemaker implantation due to medically refractory atrial tachyarrhythmias. J Interv Card Electrophysiol 1998;2(1):71–6. Available at: http://www.ncbi.nlm.nih.gov/pubmed/9869999. Accessed April 23, 2014.

61. Ganesan AN, Brooks AG, Roberts-Thomson KC, et al. Role of AV nodal ablation in cardiac resynchronization in patients with coexistent atrial fibrillation and heart failure a systematic review. J Am Coll Cardiol 2012;59(8):719–26. http://dx.doi.org/10.1016/j.jacc.2011.10.891.

62. Khan MN, Jaïs P, Cummings J, et al. Pulmonary-vein isolation for atrial fibrillation in patients with heart failure. N Engl J Med 2008;359(17):1778–85. http://dx.doi.org/10.1056/NEJMoa0708234.

63. Pappone C, Vicedomini G, Augello G, et al. Radiofrequency catheter ablation and antiarrhythmic drug therapy: a prospective, randomized, 4-year follow-up trial: the APAF study. Circ Arrhythm Electrophysiol 2011;4(6):808–14. http://dx.doi.org/10.1161/CIRCEP.111.966408.

64. Tondo C, Mantica M, Russo G, et al. Pulmonary vein vestibule ablation for the control of atrial fibrillation in patients with impaired left ventricular function. Pacing Clin Electrophysiol 2006;29(9):962–70. http://dx.doi.org/10.1111/j.1540-8159.2006.00471.x.

65. Jones DG, Haldar SK, Hussain W, et al. A randomized trial to assess catheter ablation versus rate control in the management of persistent atrial fibrillation in heart failure. J Am Coll Cardiol 2013;61(18):1894–903. http://dx.doi.org/10.1016/j.jacc.2013.01.069.

66. Hsu LF, Jaïs P, Sanders P, et al. Catheter ablation for atrial fibrillation in congestive heart failure. N Engl J Med 2004;351(23):2373–83. http://dx.doi.org/10.1056/NEJMoa041018.

67. Machino-Ohtsuka T, Seo Y, Ishizu T, et al. Efficacy, safety, and outcomes of catheter ablation of atrial fibrillation in patients with heart failure with preserved ejection fraction. J Am Coll Cardiol 2013;62(20):1857–65. http://dx.doi.org/10.1016/j.jacc.2013.07.020.

68. Myerburg RJ, Interian A, Mitrani RM, et al. Frequency of sudden cardiac death and profiles of risk. Am J Cardiol 1997;80(5B):10F–9F. Available at: http://www.ncbi.nlm.nih.gov/pubmed/9291445. Accessed April 23, 2014.

69. Myerburg RJ, Kessler KM, Castellanos A. Sudden cardiac death: epidemiology, transient risk, and intervention assessment. Ann Intern Med 1993;119(12):1187–97. Available at: http://www.ncbi.nlm.nih.gov/pubmed/8239250. Accessed April 23, 2014.

70. Huikuri HV, Castellanos A, Myerburg RJ. Sudden death due to cardiac arrhythmias. N Engl J Med

2001;345(20):1473–82. http://dx.doi.org/10.1056/NEJMra000650.

71. Effect of metoprolol CR/XL in chronic heart failure: Metoprolol CR/XL Randomised Intervention Trial in Congestive Heart Failure (MERIT-HF). Lancet 1999;353(9169):2001–7. Available at: http://www.ncbi.nlm.nih.gov/pubmed/10376614. Accessed April 9, 2014.

72. Pogwizd SM, McKenzie JP, Cain ME. Mechanisms underlying spontaneous and induced ventricular arrhythmias in patients with idiopathic dilated cardiomyopathy. Circulation 1998;98(22):2404–14. Available at: http://www.ncbi.nlm.nih.gov/pubmed/9832485. Accessed April 23, 2014.

73. Packer M, Gottlieb SS, Blum MA. Immediate and long-term pathophysiologic mechanisms underlying the genesis of sudden cardiac death in patients with congestive heart failure. Am J Med 1987; 82(3A):4–10. Available at: http://www.ncbi.nlm.nih.gov/pubmed/2882674. Accessed April 23, 2014.

74. Poole JE, Johnson GW, Hellkamp AS, et al. Prognostic importance of defibrillator shocks in patients with heart failure. N Engl J Med 2008;359(10): 1009–17. http://dx.doi.org/10.1056/NEJMoa071098.

75. Sears SF, Todaro JF, Urizar G, et al. Assessing the psychosocial impact of the ICD: a national survey of implantable cardioverter defibrillator health care providers. Pacing Clin Electrophysiol 2000;23(6): 939–45. Available at: http://www.ncbi.nlm.nih.gov/pubmed/10879376. Accessed April 23, 2014.

76. The Cardiac Insufficiency Bisoprolol Study II (CIBIS-II): a randomised trial. Lancet 1999;353(9146):9–13. Available at: http://www.ncbi.nlm.nih.gov/pubmed/10023943. Accessed April 9, 2014.

77. Packer M, Coats AJ, Fowler MB, et al. Effect of carvedilol on survival in severe chronic heart failure. N Engl J Med 2001;344(22):1651–8. http://dx.doi.org/10.1056/NEJM200105313442201.

78. Malik M, Camm AJ. Amiodarone after myocardial infarction: EMIAT and CAMIAT trials. Lancet 1997; 349(9067):1767–8. http://dx.doi.org/10.1016/S0140-6736(05)62982-0.

79. Cairns JA, Connolly SJ, Roberts R, et al. Randomised trial of outcome after myocardial infarction in patients with frequent or repetitive ventricular premature depolarisations: CAMIAT. Canadian Amiodarone Myocardial Infarction Arrhythmia Trial Investigators. Lancet 1997;349(9053):675–82. Available at: http://www.ncbi.nlm.nih.gov/pubmed/9078198. Accessed April 23, 2014.

80. Doval HC, Nul DR, Grancelli HO, et al. Randomised trial of low-dose amiodarone in severe congestive heart failure. Grupo de Estudio de la Sobrevida en la Insuficiencia Cardiaca en Argentina (GESICA). Lancet 1994;344(8921):493–8. Available at: http://www.ncbi.nlm.nih.gov/pubmed/7914611. Accessed April 23, 2014.

81. Bardy GH, Lee KL, Mark DB, et al. Amiodarone or an implantable cardioverter-defibrillator for congestive heart failure. N Engl J Med 2005;352(3):225–37. http://dx.doi.org/10.1056/NEJMoa043399.

82. Piccini JP, Berger JS, O'Connor CM. Amiodarone for the prevention of sudden cardiac death: a meta-analysis of randomized controlled trials. Eur Heart J 2009;30(10):1245–53. http://dx.doi.org/10.1093/eurheartj/ehp100.

83. Køber L, Bloch Thomsen PE, Møller M, et al. Effect of dofetilide in patients with recent myocardial infarction and left-ventricular dysfunction: a randomised trial. Lancet 2000;356(9247):2052–8. Available at: http://www.ncbi.nlm.nih.gov/pubmed/11145491. Accessed April 23, 2014.

84. Camm AJ, Karam R, Pratt CM. The azimilide post-infarct survival evaluation (ALIVE) trial. Am J Cardiol 1998;81(6A):35D–9D. Available at: http://www.ncbi.nlm.nih.gov/pubmed/9537221. Accessed April 23, 2014.

85. Callans DJ, Marchlinski FE. Dissociation of termination and prevention of inducibility of sustained ventricular tachycardia with infusion of procainamide: evidence for distinct mechanisms. J Am Coll Cardiol 1992;19(1):111–7.

86. Gorgels AP, van den Dool A, Hofs A, et al. Comparison of procainamide and lidocaine in terminating sustained monomorphic ventricular tachycardia. Am J Cardiol 1996;78(1):43–6.

87. Sharma AD, Purves P, Yee R, et al. Hemodynamic effects of intravenous procainamide during ventricular tachycardia. Am Heart J 1990;119(5): 1034–41.

88. Kułakowski P, Karczmarewicz S, Karpiński G, et al. Effects of intravenous amiodarone on ventricular refractoriness, intraventricular conduction, and ventricular tachycardia induction. Europace 2000; 2(3):207–15. http://dx.doi.org/10.1053/eupc.2000.0099.

89. Mitchell LB, Wyse DG, Gillis AM, et al. Electropharmacology of amiodarone therapy initiation. Time courses of onset of electrophysiologic and antiarrhythmic effects. Circulation 1989; 80(1):34–42.

90. Nademanee K, Taylor R, Bailey WE, et al. Treating electrical storm: sympathetic blockade versus advanced cardiac life support-guided therapy. Circulation 2000;102(7):742–7.

91. Moss AJ, Zareba W, Hall WJ, et al. Prophylactic implantation of a defibrillator in patients with myocardial infarction and reduced ejection fraction. N Engl J Med 2002;346(12):877–83. http://dx.doi.org/10.1056/NEJMoa013474.

92. Pacifico A, Hohnloser SH, Williams JH, et al. Prevention of implantable-defibrillator shocks by treatment with sotalol. d,l-Sotalol Implantable Cardioverter-Defibrillator Study Group. N Engl J

Med 1999;340(24):1855–62. http://dx.doi.org/10.1056/NEJM199906173402402.

93. Singer I, Al-Khalidi H, Niazi I, et al. Azimilide decreases recurrent ventricular tachyarrhythmias in patients with implantable cardioverter defibrillators. J Am Coll Cardiol 2004;43(1):39–43. Available at: http://www.ncbi.nlm.nih.gov/pubmed/14715180. Accessed April 23, 2014.

94. Connolly SJ, Dorian P, Roberts RS, et al. Comparison of beta-blockers, amiodarone plus beta-blockers, or sotalol for prevention of shocks from implantable cardioverter defibrillators: the OPTIC Study: a randomized trial. JAMA 2006;295(2):165–71. http://dx.doi.org/10.1001/jama.295.2.165.

95. Hohnloser SH, Dorian P, Roberts R, et al. Effect of amiodarone and sotalol on ventricular defibrillation threshold: the Optimal Pharmacological Therapy in Cardioverter Defibrillator Patients (OPTIC) trial. Circulation 2006;114(2):104–9. http://dx.doi.org/10.1161/CIRCULATIONAHA.106.618421.

The Role of Heart Failure Pharmacotherapy After Left Ventricular Assist Device Support

CrossMark

John J. Rommel, MD, Thomas J. O'Neill, MD, PhD,
Anton Lishmanov, MD, PhD, Jason N. Katz, MD, MHS,
Patricia P. Chang, MD, MHS*

KEYWORDS

- Left ventricular assist device • Mechanical circulatory support • Heart failure • Medical therapy
- Review

KEY POINTS

- Left ventricular assist device (LVAD) implantation is becoming more common for the management of end-stage heart failure.
- Very few evidence-based studies on optimal medical therapy post-LVAD exist, and treatment often varies across institutions.
- In select patient populations, aggressive heart failure medical therapy after LVAD implantation may reduce cardiac remodeling, improve biventricular function, and possibly promote left ventricular recovery.
- Future investigations are needed to confirm which patients will benefit from aggressive medical therapy after LVAD implantation.

INTRODUCTION

Mechanical circulatory support has been in existence since the 1960s. Since approval by the Food and Drug Administration of a pneumatically driven left ventricular assist device (LVAD) as bridge to transplant in 1994 and as destination therapy in 2002, and with newer continuous-flow and centrifugal devices, LVADs have become an increasingly frequent treatment option for patients with end-stage heart failure. As of early 2013, The Interagency Registry for Mechanically Assisted Circulatory Support (INTERMACS) has 7900 LVADs in their registry, of which approximately 6000 were implanted since 2010.[1]

Given this rapidly expanding treatment option, our understanding of how to best manage LVAD patients pharmacologically is also evolving. In general, pharmacotherapy after LVAD support is directed at the following goals: (1) antithrombotic agents to prevent LVAD pump and aortic root thrombosis; (2) antihypertensives to control systemic blood pressure and left ventricular (LV) afterload; (3) heart failure–specific therapies to reverse LV remodeling, support right ventricular (RV) function, and enhance biventricular recovery; (4) diuretics to prevent volume overload; and (5) antiarrhythmics to prevent or control arrhythmias.

Disclosure Statement: The authors have no relevant conflict of interests to disclose.
Division of Cardiology, Department of Medicine, The University of North Carolina at Chapel Hill, 160 Dental Circle, 6th Floor Burnett-Womack Building, Chapel Hill, NC 27599-7075, USA
* Corresponding author.
E-mail address: patricia_chang@med.unc.edu

Heart Failure Clin 10 (2014) 653–660
http://dx.doi.org/10.1016/j.hfc.2014.07.008
1551-7136/14/$ – see front matter © 2014 Elsevier Inc. All rights reserved.

heartfailure.theclinics.com

At present, maintaining patients on evidence-based heart failure therapies after LVAD implantation varies across institutions. This variability probably depends on the goal of LVAD support, whether for destination therapy, bridge to transplant, or bridge to myocardial recovery. For example, in one study of 20 patients with LVADs as a bridge to transplant, only 5% were on β-blockers, 35% on angiotensin-converting enzyme inhibitors (ACEIs), and 20% on diuretics[2]; whereas in a second study of 28 patients, of whom 75% received LVAD as destination therapy, more than 50% of LVAD recipients were on β-blockers.[3] The International Society for Heart and Lung Transplant (ISHLT) guidelines for mechanical circulatory support provide only brief recommendations on chronic heart failure therapy, all of which are derived from expert opinion.[4] The goal of this article is to review the current literature and guidelines for heart failure–specific pharmacotherapy in the LVAD patient, and explore future treatment possibilities. **Table 1** summarizes these therapies by pharmacologic class and the recommendations

regarding their use in patients supported with an LVAD.

ANGIOTENSIN-CONVERTING ENZYME INHIBITORS/ANGIOTENSIN II RECEPTOR BLOCKERS

ACEIs and angiotensin II receptor blockers (ARBs) are well established in the medical management of patients with systolic heart failure.[5] However, the current ISHLT guidelines for mechanical circulatory support recommend the use of ACEIs and ARBs only for management of hypertension and cardiovascular risk reduction in patients with diabetes and vascular disease (Class I, level of evidence C).[4] Despite the limited recommendations, these medications may provide further benefit.

Although data are limited, patients can have improved LV contractile function after LVAD placement with the use of an ACEI or ARB. Klotz and colleagues[6] evaluated the effects of concomitant angiotensin inhibition during pulsatile LVAD support by retrospectively comparing 7 patients

Table 1
Management of heart failure in the LVAD patient by pharmacologic class

Medication	Recommendation[a]/Goals	Class[a]	Level of Evidence[a]
ACEIs/ARBs	For hypertension	I	C
	For risk reduction in vascular disease and diabetes	I	C
	Protective effects from remodeling	—	—
Aldosterone antagonists	To limit need for potassium repletion	I	C
	Potential antifibrotic effects	I	C
β-blockers	For hypertension	I	C
	For rate control for tachyarrhythmias	I	C
	May be useful in the setting of current VT	IIa	C
Hydralazine	For hypertension	I	C
Nitrates	For hypertension	I	C
Clenbuterol	May help LV recovery for LVAD explantation	—	—
Digoxin	May be useful in the setting of atrial fibrillation with rapid ventricular response	II	C
	Could be useful to improve RV dysfunction	—	—
Diuretics	For management of volume overload	I	C
	For management of RV dysfunction	I	C
Inotropes	For management of RV dysfunction	I	C
PDE-5 inhibitors	May be useful for management of RV dysfunction in the setting of pulmonary arterial hypertension	IIb	C
Endothelin receptor antagonists	Can be considered for additional management of RV dysfunction in the setting of pulmonary arterial hypertension	—	—

Abbreviations: ACEI, angiotensin-converting enzyme inhibitor; ARB, angiotensin II receptor blocker; LV, left ventricular; PDE-5, phosphodiesterase-5; RV, right ventricular; VT, ventricular tachycardia.
[a] Based on the 2013 International Society for Heart and Lung Transplantation Guidelines for mechanical circulatory support: executive summary.[4]

receiving an ACEI while on LVAD support with 15 LVAD patients who were not receiving an ACEI. This medical therapy was associated with decreased LV mass and stiffness during LVAD support. As also discussed in the article in this issue by Reed and colleagues and elsewhere, ACEI and ARB use results in reverse LV remodeling probably by inhibiting the renin-angiotensin-aldosterone system (RAAS), resulting in prevention of myocardial fibrosis and a reduced extracellular collagen matrix (ECM).[7]

Mechanical LV unloading with the LVAD also results in significant reversal of remodeling with improved hemodynamics, reduced LV chamber size, reduced LV mass, and myocyte function.[8,9] However, ECM remodeling is not reversed during mechanical unloading and, instead, LVAD support may modify ECM in a potentially detrimental way. For this reason, ACEIs may be beneficial for LVAD recipients. In a study of 16 patients supported with a pulsatile LVAD as a bridge to transplant, explanted hearts demonstrated increased collagen deposition, increased collagen cross-linking, increased myocardial stiffness, and increased tissue angiotensin II.[10] When cardiac neurohormones were measured in 2 other case series of patients who were supported with an LVAD before transplant, mechanical LV unloading was associated with higher levels of cardiac angiotensin II[6] and a 7-fold increase in cardiac norepinephrine.[11] However, explanted hearts from patients who were on ACEIs while on LVAD support demonstrated a decrease in angiotensin II levels[6] and no increase in norepinephrine levels.[11]

Some insight into the disease-modifying properties of ACEIs is suggested in other observational studies reporting the rate of successful LVAD explantation. Studies reporting 100% use of ACEIs had higher rates of cardiac recovery, such as 24%[12] and 38%[13] of the LVAD-supported patients. In studies where fewer ACEIs were used, there were lower rates of improvement in LV contractility. For example, in the case series by Maybaum and colleagues,[14] 27% of patients received ACEIs and only 6% achieved cardiac recovery sufficient for LVAD removal. In another series by Sun and colleagues[15] in which none of the patients supported with LVAD received ACEIs or any neurohormonal-targeted therapy, the reported rate of explantation was only 4%. However, it should be noted that these studies varied greatly and contained many other variables beyond ACEI use.

Overall RAAS inhibition is associated with favorable effects on reverse remodeling in LVAD patients, primarily because of a decrease in the ECM and fibrosis.[7] Strategies of targeting RAAS in patients with LVADs need more investigation, but should be considered in all LVAD patients who do not have contraindications.

ALDOSTERONE ANTAGONISTS

Also acting in the RAAS pathway, excess aldosterone is known to contribute to pathologic cardiomyocyte remodeling and expansion of fibrosis.[7] Although no studies have specifically examined the benefits of aldosterone antagonists in LVAD recipients, Klotz and colleagues[6] demonstrated that elevated aldosterone levels persist in LVAD patients even in the setting of ACEI. These potential beneficial effects are the reason why low-dose spironolactone has been a component of protocols used for bridging to cardiac recovery and explantation of LVAD in nonischemic cardiomyopathy patients.[16] Aldosterone antagonists also promote salt excretion while inhibiting potassium excretion. This additional effect makes these medications useful in patients who continue to require moderate doses of loop diuretics or potassium supplementation after LVAD implantation. As a result of these data, the ISHLT has classified aldosterone antagonist use as a Class I recommendation for its potential antifibrotic and potassium-sparing effects.[4]

β-BLOCKERS

In the current ISHLT guidelines, β-blockers also have a Class I indication for the treatment of hypertension and tachyarrhythmias in addition to a Class IIa indication for the treatment of recurrent ventricular tachycardia.[4] However, these recommendations attain a level of evidence C. Nevertheless, there are some data to suggest that β-blockers are useful in the LVAD population in halting or even reversing pathologic LV remodeling. Given their effect on the sympathetic system, β-blockers have been part of pharmacologic treatment protocols used to improve LV function for possible LVAD explantation.[16,17] In addition, not starting a β-blocker in the postoperative period after LVAD implantation has been found to be the strongest predictor of ventricular arrhythmias.[18] Unfortunately, many of these studies are small and retrospective, and it is difficult to draw significant conclusions from them. Given the known benefits of β-blockers in the general systolic heart failure population, using them after LVAD implantation is appropriate when the patient is hemodynamically stable and euvolemic, especially if there are coexisting arrhythmias and hypertension, or hope for LV recovery.

DIGOXIN

Digoxin is another historical mainstay in the management of heart failure, with evidence of improved cardiac output, symptomatic benefit, and decreased hospital admissions for heart failure. Yet digoxin has never been associated with mortality benefit in the heart failure population.[19] Furthermore, more recent data have also cast doubt on any potential benefit of digoxin in advanced heart failure. Georgiopoulou and colleagues[20] performed a retrospective review of 455 patients with end-stage heart failure, half of whom were on digoxin and were at higher risk for the primary outcomes of death, urgent transplant, or LVAD implantation. Based on the current literature, digoxin has a Class II indication in the ISHLT guidelines only for LVAD patients with atrial fibrillation who require rate control.[4]

However, digoxin may be beneficial in isolated RV failure resulting from severe pulmonary hypertension. Acute digoxin loading has been shown to improve RV function as assessed by invasive hemodynamic measures.[21] More recently, Eshtehardi and colleagues[22] reported that digoxin therapy may provide a mortality benefit in this patient population. Though interesting, it remains unclear whether these findings can be replicated in the subset of LVAD patients who develop or continue to have significant RV failure after LVAD implantation. Nevertheless, digoxin has been incorporated into bridge-to-recovery strategies aimed at eventual LVAD removal.[23] Overall, digoxin is probably best used as a second-line medication for those with atrial arrhythmias or significant RV failure, or with goals for myocardial recovery.

DIURETICS

Diuretics, particularly loop diuretics, are almost universally required to maintain normal fluid balance before LVAD implantation.[24] Following mechanical LV unloading with improvements in cardiac output and filling pressures, diuretic dosage generally decreases after LVAD implantation. In many cases, standing loop diuretics can be completely eliminated. In one case series, only 4 of 20 (20%) LVAD patients were taking diuretics at the time of transplant.[2] As there is no evidence that loop diuretics improve long-term outcomes in patients with heart failure with or without mechanical circulatory support, routine use of diuretics post-LVAD should be only used when necessary to maintain euvolemia. In fact, overdiuresis can lead to underfilling of the left ventricle, causing LVAD-related suction events and ventricular arrhythmias. Patients with chronic RV dysfunction are more likely to require diuretics to avoid central venous congestion and subsequent renal and hepatic dysfunction.[25] Thiazide diuretics can also be used to augment diuresis when loop diuretics are insufficient. Diuretics are a reasonable component of post-LVAD medical therapy and are a Class I indication in the ISHLT guidelines, but are ideally used at the lowest doses needed to achieve symptomatic relief.[4]

THERAPIES FOR PULMONARY HYPERTENSION

RV dysfunction after LVAD surgery is associated with worse outcomes.[25] Pre-LVAD RV dysfunction often does not improve after LV mechanical unloading and, in fact, may worsen.[26] Although chronic LVAD support is associated with improved transpulmonary pressure gradients over time, this may take months to occur.[27] Persistently elevated pulmonary vascular resistance (PVR) is associated with post-LVAD RV failure. Inhaled nitric oxide[28] and iloprost[29] have been demonstrated to improve pulmonary artery pressures and increase LVAD flows in cases of elevated PVR and RV dysfunction. Although these therapies have been primarily used in the immediate postoperative setting, specifically treating markedly elevated PVR in LVAD patients with long-term therapy is often necessary to avoid further RV failure. Phosphodiesterase-5 (PDE-5) inhibitors, such as sildenafil, have been shown to improve hemodynamics[30] and exercise capacity[31] in patients with pulmonary hypertension caused by left heart failure without LVADs. In an open-label study of LVAD recipients, sildenafil therapy plus LVAD support was more effective than LVAD alone in lowering PVR.[32]

Beyond PDE-5 inhibitors, there are some reports of success in improving pulmonary hypertension with endothelin receptor antagonists such as bosentan.[33] One single-center case series looked at 50 patients on bosentan and found the drug to be well tolerated in their LVAD population. In addition, at 6-month follow-up there was right-sided decongestion with improvement in both the bilirubin and alkaline phosphatase levels.[34] Thus, for patients with RV dysfunction and pulmonary hypertension, PDE-5 inhibitors are a Class IIb indication.[4] Although endothelin receptor antagonists are not specifically mentioned in the current ISHLT guidelines, these medications can also be considered to treat persistent post-LVAD right heart failure related to high PVR, but should probably be considered a second-line therapy.

CLENBUTEROL

Clenbuterol is a β2-agonist and is one of the few drugs that has been specifically evaluated in the LVAD patient population. In 2006, Birks and colleagues[17] published a study showing that 11 of 15 patients with pulsatile LVADs were able to undergo LVAD explantation, owing to sufficient myocardial recovery. The study protocol used a combination of evidence-based heart failure therapies (lisinopril, carvedilol, spironolactone, and losartan) in addition to clenbuterol.[17] This study was followed by a second similar one published in 2011 involving 20 nonischemic patients on continuous-flow LVADs.[16] In the second study, the patients were started on a combination of lisinopril, losartan, carvedilol, spironolactone, and digoxin. These medications were titrated to the maximum treatment dose or maximally tolerated dose. Once the LV diameter had decreased sufficiently (to allow for maximum LV unloading), carvedilol was changed to a β1-selective antagonist (bisoprolol) and clenbuterol added. The investigators found that 12 of the 20 patients had recovery of their left ventricle and underwent LVAD explantation after 286 ± 97 days of support. Although 2 of the 12 patients died shortly after explantation, the 30-day, 1-year, and 3-year survival without recurrence of heart failure was 83.3%. The investigators suggested that one possible explanation for such results was that the LVAD allowed the patient to tolerate more heart failure therapy than before LVAD implantation, which prevented and reversed pathologic remodeling. In addition, clenbuterol created a state of "physiologic hypertrophy," which may have improved ventricular function.[16] These results were more impressive than those of other studies, which found significantly lower results of LV recovery, ranging from less than 1% to 24%.[12] Nevertheless, it remains unclear from the studies by Birks and colleagues[16,17] how much of the improvement came from clenbuterol. It is noteworthy that LV systolic function had normalized in these patients before the addition of clenbuterol, and that this study was not placebo controlled.[35] In addition, many of these patients were younger and had not been in systolic heart failure for a long period of time. Furthermore, preliminary results from a larger, multicenter trial involving clenbuterol have not shown the same results.[36] At present, clenbuterol is not mentioned in the ISHLT guidelines for mechanical circulatory support and is currently not approved in the United States for human use.

INOTROPES

Overall there is very little evidence to guide the use of inotropes in patients with LVADs. The most common reason for using inotropic therapy in a patient supported with an LVAD is right heart failure. Postoperatively, inotropic support is usually weaned within the first 2 weeks. However, the rate of weaning inotrope therapy depends on the individual patient's degree of RV dysfunction. In previous studies the prevalence of RV dysfunction requiring inotropic support 30 days after LVAD implantation was 3.75%[37] and 2.8%,[38] respectively. One small case report suggests that milrinone may have some advantage in this setting in comparison with dobutamine, as it is both an inotropic agent and a pulmonary vasodilator.[39] There are no available data describing long-term survival in the rare cases where chronic inotrope therapy is needed in the LVAD destination therapy patient. Nevertheless, although no specific medications are named, the use of inotropes in the setting of RV dysfunction in an LVAD patient has received a Class I indication in the current ISHLT guidelines.[4]

MANAGEMENT OF HYPERTENSION

Although elevated blood pressures are rarely an issue in the pre-LVAD heart failure population, improved cardiac output with LVAD support often results in either normal blood pressure or some degree of hypertension postoperatively. Elevated blood pressure can impair mechanical unloading of the left ventricle and can increase the risk of aortic insufficiency, aortic root thrombosis, pump malfunction, and neurovascular events.[40] Continuous-flow LVADs are more sensitive to elevated blood pressure then pulsatile pumps because elevated afterload decreases the pressure gradient across the pump, leading to less pump flow and less effective mechanical unloading.[41] Newer-generation centrifugal pumps appear to be even more sensitive to elevated blood pressure than axial flow pumps.[41]

No studies to date have associated clinical outcomes with specific blood pressure targets, so the basis for guidelines is somewhat empiric and is based on consensus opinion. Recommendations vary but often suggest a goal mean arterial pressure (MAP) of between 65 and 80 mm Hg, with more aggressive treatment for MAP greater than 90 mm Hg.[42,43] The current ISHLT guidelines suggest that nonpulsatile devices should have a MAP goal of 80 mm Hg or less (Class IIb indication).[4] The preferred mechanism for treating blood pressure in LVAD patients is by reduction of systemic vascular resistance and avoidance of negative inotropic agents. Given their effects on afterload reduction and blockade of the RAAS systems, ACEIs or ARBs should be first-line therapy for hypertensive LVAD patients, followed by β-blockers.

Other antihypertensive agents often used for heart failure, such as hydralazine and nitrates, should also be considered as needed. All of these heart failure medications have a Class I indication in the ISHLT guidelines.[4]

SUMMARY

Overall much investigation is still needed to better understand what would constitute optimal medical heart failure therapy in patients with LVADs. Almost all classes of heart failure medication would benefit from dedicated studies looking at their role in the LVAD patient population, this being especially true for those patients whose LVAD support is considered to be a potential bridge to recovery. Although the studies by Birks and colleagues[16,17] offer the interesting possibility of reversing end-stage heart failure in select patients with pharmacotherapy after LVAD implantation, it is important to continue to define which patients might benefit from an aggressive medical strategy. In addition, further studies are needed to evaluate the benefits of these medications beyond recovery of LV contractile function.

Current heart failure medications such as ACEIs, ARBs, β-blockers, aldosterone antagonists, digoxin, and diuretics should be considered in patients with LVADs, depending on comorbidities and the specific goal of LVAD support for individual patients (see **Table 1**). Controlling hypertension should be a priority in all patients with nonpulsatile LVADs, and is associated with better outcomes such as decreased rate of stroke. In addition, comorbid conditions such as coronary artery disease and tachyarrhythmias should be treated with evidence-based therapies that have been validated in the general heart failure population without LVADs. For those with persistent pulmonary hypertension post-LVAD, the use of PDE-5 inhibitors and/or endothelin receptor antagonists can prevent further RV dysfunction. However, if LV recovery is not the goal and until more investigation is done, there is equipoise regarding whether aggressive heart failure pharmacotherapy should be continued at target doses or even pursued post LVAD. Appropriate use of these medications should be considered on an individualized basis.

REFERENCES

1. Kirklin JK, Naftel DC, Kormos RL, et al. Third INTERMACS annual report: the evolution of destination therapy in the United States. J Heart Lung Transplant 2011;30(2):115–23. http://dx.doi.org/10.1016/j.healun.2010.12.001.

2. Ambardekar AV, Buttrick PM. Reverse remodeling with left ventricular assist devices: a review of clinical, cellular, and molecular effects. Circ Heart Fail 2011;4(2):224–33. http://dx.doi.org/10.1161/CIRCHEARTFAILURE.110.959684.

3. Jennings DL, Jones MC, Lanfear DE. Assessment of the heart failure pharmacotherapy of patients with continuous flow left-ventricular assist devices. Int J Artif Organs 2012;35(3):177–9. http://dx.doi.org/10.5301/ijao.5000068.

4. Feldman D, Pamboukian SV, Teuteberg JJ, et al. The 2013 international society for heart and lung transplantation guidelines for mechanical circulatory support: executive summary. J Heart Lung Transplant 2013;32(2):157–87. http://dx.doi.org/10.1016/j.healun.2012.09.013.

5. Yancy CW, Jessup M, Bozkurt B, et al. 2013 ACCF/AHA guideline for the management of heart failure: a report of the American College of Cardiology Foundation/American Heart Association task force on practice guidelines. J Am Coll Cardiol 2013;62(16):e147–239. http://dx.doi.org/10.1016/j.jacc.2013.05.019.

6. Klotz S, Danser AH, Foronjy RF, et al. The impact of angiotensin-converting enzyme inhibitor therapy on the extracellular collagen matrix during left ventricular assist device support in patients with end-stage heart failure. J Am Coll Cardiol 2007;49(11):1166–74.

7. Jugdutt BI. Remodeling of the myocardium and potential targets in the collagen degradation and synthesis pathways. Curr Drug Targets Cardiovasc Haematol Disord 2003;3(1):1–30.

8. Burkhoff D, Klotz S, Mancini DM. LVAD-induced reverse remodeling: basic and clinical implications for myocardial recovery. J Card Fail 2006;12(3):227–39.

9. Butler CR, Jugdutt BI. The paradox of left ventricular assist device unloading and myocardial recovery in end-stage dilated cardiomyopathy: implications for heart failure in the elderly. Heart Fail Rev 2012;17(4–5):615–33. http://dx.doi.org/10.1007/s10741-012-9300-8.

10. Klotz S, Foronjy RF, Dickstein ML, et al. Mechanical unloading during left ventricular assist device support increases left ventricular collagen cross-linking and myocardial stiffness. Circulation 2005;112(3):364–74.

11. Klotz S, Burkhoff D, Garrelds IM, et al. The impact of left ventricular assist device-induced left ventricular unloading on the myocardial renin-angiotensin-aldosterone system: therapeutic consequences? Eur Heart J 2009;30(7):805–12. http://dx.doi.org/10.1093/eurheartj/ehp012.

12. Dandel M, Weng Y, Siniawski H, et al. Heart failure reversal by ventricular unloading in patients with chronic cardiomyopathy: criteria for weaning from ventricular assist devices. Eur Heart J 2011;32(9):1148–60. http://dx.doi.org/10.1093/eurheartj/ehq353.

13. Matsumiya G, Monta O, Fukushima N, et al. Who would be a candidate for bridge to recovery during prolonged mechanical left ventricular support in idiopathic dilated cardiomyopathy? J Thorac Cardiovasc Surg 2005;130(3):699–704.

14. Maybaum S, Mancini D, Xydas S, et al. Cardiac improvement during mechanical circulatory support: a prospective multicenter study of the LVAD working group. Circulation 2007;115(19):2497–505.

15. Sun BC, Catanese KA, Spanier TB, et al. 100 long-term implantable left ventricular assist devices: the Columbia Presbyterian interim experience. Ann Thorac Surg 1999;68(2):688–94.

16. Birks EJ, George RS, Hedger M, et al. Reversal of severe heart failure with a continuous-flow left ventricular assist device and pharmacological therapy: a prospective study. Circulation 2011;123(4):381–90. http://dx.doi.org/10.1161/CIRCULATIONAHA.109.933960.

17. Birks EJ, Tansley PD, Hardy J, et al. Left ventricular assist device and drug therapy for the reversal of heart failure. N Engl J Med 2006;355(18):1873–84.

18. Refaat M, Chemaly E, Lebeche D, et al. Ventricular arrhythmias after left ventricular assist device implantation. Pacing Clin Electrophysiol 2008; 31(10):1246–52. http://dx.doi.org/10.1111/j.1540-8159.2008.01173.x.

19. Gheorghiade M, Adams KF Jr, Colucci WS. Digoxin in the management of cardiovascular disorders. Circulation 2004;109(24):2959–64. http://dx.doi.org/10.1161/01.CIR.0000132482.95686.87.

20. Georgiopoulou VV, Kalogeropoulos AP, Giamouzis G, et al. Digoxin therapy does not improve outcomes in patients with advanced heart failure on contemporary medical therapy. Circ Heart Fail 2009;2(2):90–7. http://dx.doi.org/10.1161/CIRCHEARTFAILURE.108.807032.

21. Rich S, Seidlitz M, Dodin E, et al. The short-term effects of digoxin in patients with right ventricular dysfunction from pulmonary hypertension. Chest 1998;114(3):787–92.

22. Eshtehardi P, Mojadidi M, Khosraviani K, et al. Effect of digoxin on mortality in patients with isolated right ventricular dysfunction secondary to severe pulmonary hypertension. J Am Coll Cardiol 2014;63(12S). http://dx.doi.org/10.1016/S0735-1097(14)60750-6.

23. Lenneman AJ, Birks EJ. Treatment strategies for myocardial recovery in heart failure. Curr Treat Options Cardiovasc Med 2014;16(3):287. http://dx.doi.org/10.1007/s11936-013-0287-9.

24. McDiarmid A, Gordon B, Wrightson N, et al. Hemodynamic, echocardiographic, and exercise-related effects of the HeartWare left ventricular assist device in advanced heart failure. Congest Heart Fail 2013;19(1):11–5. http://dx.doi.org/10.1111/j.1751-7133.2012.00302.x.

25. Patlolla B, Beygui R, Haddad F. Right-ventricular failure following left ventricle assist device implantation.

26. Palardy M, Nohria A, Rivero J, et al. Right ventricular dysfunction during intensive pharmacologic unloading persists after mechanical unloading. J Card Fail 2010;16(3):218–24. http://dx.doi.org/10.1016/j.cardfail.2009.11.002.

27. Mikus E, Stepanenko A, Krabatsch T, et al. Reversibility of fixed pulmonary hypertension in left ventricular assist device support recipients. Eur J Cardiothorac Surg 2011;40(4):971–7. http://dx.doi.org/10.1016/j.ejcts.2011.01.019.

28. Argenziano M, Choudhri AF, Moazami N, et al. Randomized, double-blind trial of inhaled nitric oxide in LVAD recipients with pulmonary hypertension. Ann Thorac Surg 1998;65(2):340–5.

29. Antoniou T, Prokakis C, Athanasopoulos G, et al. Inhaled nitric oxide plus iloprost in the setting of post-left assist device right heart dysfunction. Ann Thorac Surg 2012;94(3):792–8. http://dx.doi.org/10.1016/j.athoracsur.2012.04.046.

30. Lepore JJ, Maroo A, Bigatello LM, et al. Hemodynamic effects of sildenafil in patients with congestive heart failure and pulmonary hypertension: combined administration with inhaled nitric oxide. Chest 2005;127(5):1647–53. http://dx.doi.org/10.1378/chest.127.5.1647.

31. Lewis GD, Shah R, Shahzad K, et al. Sildenafil improves exercise capacity and quality of life in patients with systolic heart failure and secondary pulmonary hypertension. Circulation 2007;116(14):1555–62.

32. Tedford RJ, Hemnes AR, Russell SD, et al. PDE5A inhibitor treatment of persistent pulmonary hypertension after mechanical circulatory support. Circ Heart Fail 2008;1(4):213–9. http://dx.doi.org/10.1161/CIRCHEARTFAILURE.108.796789.

33. Imamura T, Kinugawa K, Hatano M, et al. Bosentan improved persistent pulmonary hypertension in a case after implantation of a left ventricular assist device. J Artif Organs 2013;16(1):101–4. http://dx.doi.org/10.1007/s10047-012-0662-4.

34. LaRue SJ, Garcia-Cortes R, Ray S, et al. Treatment of secondary pulmonary hypertension with bosentan after left ventricular assist device implantation. J Heart Lung Transplant 2013;32(4 Suppl):S110. http://dx.doi.org/10.1016/j.healun.2013.01.228.

35. Maybaum S. Cardiac recovery during continuous-flow left ventricular assist device support: some good news from across the Atlantic. Circulation 2011;123(4):355–7. http://dx.doi.org/10.1161/CIRCULATIONAHA.110.005199.

36. Abstracts of the International Society for Heart and Lung Transplantation Thirty-First Annual Meeting and Scientific Sessions. April 13-16, 2011. San Diego, California, USA. J Heart Lung Transplant 2011;30(4 Suppl):S8–228.

Curr Opin Cardiol 2013;28(2):223–33. http://dx.doi.org/10.1097/HCO.0b013e32835dd12c.

37. Miller LW, Pagani FD, Russell SD, et al. Use of a continuous-flow device in patients awaiting heart transplantation. N Engl J Med 2007;357(9):885–96.

38. Pagani FD, Miller LW, Russell SD, et al. Extended mechanical circulatory support with a continuous-flow rotary left ventricular assist device. J Am Coll Cardiol 2009;54(4):312–21. http://dx.doi.org/10.1016/j.jacc.2009.03.055.

39. Kihara S, Kawai A, Fukuda T, et al. Effects of milrinone for right ventricular failure after left ventricular assist device implantation. Heart Vessels 2002;16(2):69–71.

40. Slaughter MS, Pagani FD, Rogers JG, et al. Clinical management of continuous-flow left ventricular assist devices in advanced heart failure. J Heart Lung Transplant 2010;29(4 Suppl):S1–39. http://dx.doi.org/10.1016/j.healun.2010.01.011.

41. Lampert BC, Eckert C, Weaver S, et al. Blood pressure control in continuous flow left ventricular assist devices: efficacy and impact on adverse events. Ann Thorac Surg 2014;97(1):139–46. http://dx.doi.org/10.1016/j.athoracsur.2013.07.069.

42. John R, Kamdar F, Eckman P, et al. Lessons learned from experience with over 100 consecutive HeartMate II left ventricular assist devices. Ann Thorac Surg 2011;92(5):1593–9. http://dx.doi.org/10.1016/j.athoracsur.2011.06.081 [discussion: 1599–600].

43. Myers TJ, Bolmers M, Gregoric ID, et al. Assessment of arterial blood pressure during support with an axial flow left ventricular assist device. J Heart Lung Transplant 2009;28(5):423–7. http://dx.doi.org/10.1016/j.healun.2009.01.013.

Index

Note: Page numbers of article titles are in **boldface** type.

A

African-American Heart Failure Trial - 2004, 567–568

Aldosterone, role in heart failure, 560–561

Aldosterone antagonists, and left ventricular assist device recipients, 655
in heart failure, 571

Aldosterone escape, 550–551

Aldosterone receptor antagonist(s), in heart failure with reduced ejection fraction, 595
reverse remodeling and, 550

Aldosterone synthase inhibitors, 562–563

Aliskiren, in heart failure with reduced ejection fraction, 579

Amiodarone, in heart failure, 639–642, 644, 645

Anemia, and iron deficiency, in heart failure, drugs used in, 582

Angiotensin-converting enzyme inhibitors, and hemodynamics of heart failure, 550, 559
antiarrhythmic effects of, 550
escape, 550–551
in heart failure with reduced ejection fraction, 578, 593

Angiotensin-converting enzyme inhibitors/angiotensin II receptor blockers, in systolic heart failure, 654–655

Angiotensin receptor blocker, in heart failure with reduced ejection fraction, 578, 593

Antiarrhythmic drug therapy, for prevention of shocks by implantable cardioverter defibrillators, 646–647
for prophylaxis of ventricular arrhythmia in heart failure, 643–645

Antiarrhythmic drugs, membrane active, 639, 640–641
mode of action of, 636, 644

Antiarrhythmic therapy, current approaches to, in heart failure, **635–652**

Anticoagulant therapy, in heart failure with comorbidities, 579–581

Anticoagulants, novel oral, compared, 580

Antiplatelet therapy, in heart failure with comorbidities, 579–581

Arrhythmia(s), supraventricular, 635
ventricular. See *Ventricular arrhythmias.*

Arthritis, and gout, in heart failure, drugs used in, 582

Atherosclerosis, in heart failure, 622

Atorvastatin, in heart failure, 629, 630, 631, 632

Atrial fibrillation, and heart failure, 636–637
catheter ablation in, 642–643

epidemiology and pathophysiology of, 635–637
rate control in, 639–642
rhythm control in, 639
with heart failure, acute management of, 637
long-term management of, 637
rhythm control in, 637–638
nonpharmacologic approaches to, 642–643

Azimilide, in heart failure, 645

B

ß-Blockers, and molecular changes in human heart, 547
antiarrhythmic effects of, 547
benefit in human heart, mechanisms of, 546–548
hemodynamics of, 546–547
in heart failure, 601, 639, 644, 646, 655
in heart failure with reduced ejection fraction, 578, 593–595
use in ventricular remodeling, 547
used in heart failure trials, classification and effects of, 546

C

Calcium channel blockers, in heart failure, 639

Canrenone, in heart failure clinical trials, 561

Cardiovascular physiology, renin-angiotensin-aldosterone system and, 548, 549
sympathetic nervous system and, 544

Carvedilol, in heart failure, 571, 644

Catheter ablation, in atrial fibrillation, 642–643

Cholesterol levels, in heart failure, 622

Clenbuterol, in left ventricular assist device patients, 657

Conivaptan, 607, 610–611

D

Defibrillators, implantable cardioverter, shocks by, antiarrhythmic drugs for prevention of, 646–647

Depression, in heart failure, drugs used in, 582

Diabetes mellitus, in heart failure, drugs used in, 581

Digoxin, and sympathetic nervous system, 547–548
in heart failure, 639, 656

Diuretics, and antialdosterone effects of mineralcorticoid receptor agonists, resistance to, 561

Heart Failure Clin 10 (2014) 661–664
http://dx.doi.org/10.1016/S1551-7136(14)00078-6
1551-7136/14/$ – see front matter © 2014 Elsevier Inc. All rights reserved.

United States Postal Service

Statement of Ownership, Management, and Circulation
(All Periodicals Publications Except Requestor Publications)

1. Publication Title	2. Publication Number	3. Filing Date
Heart Failure Clinics	0 2 5 - 0 5 5	9/14/14

4. Issue Frequency	5. Number of Issues Published Annually	6. Annual Subscription Price
Jan, Apr, Jul, Oct	4	$235.00

7. Complete Mailing Address of Known Office of Publication (Not printer) (Street, city, county, state, and ZIP+4®)

Elsevier Inc.
360 Park Avenue South
New York, NY 10010-1710

Contact Person
Stephen R. Bushing
Telephone (Include area code)
215-239-3688

8. Complete Mailing Address of Headquarters or General Business Office of Publisher (Not printer)

Elsevier Inc., 360 Park Avenue South, New York, NY 10010-1710

9. Full Names and Complete Mailing Addresses of Publisher, Editor, and Managing Editor (Do not leave blank)

Publisher (Name and complete mailing address)

Linda Belfus, Elsevier Inc., 1600 John F. Kennedy Blvd., Suite 1800, Philadelphia, PA 19103-2899

Editor (Name and complete mailing address)

Adrianne Brigido, Elsevier Inc., 1600 John F. Kennedy Blvd., Suite 1800, Philadelphia, PA 19103-2899

Managing Editor (Name and complete mailing address)

Mary Gatsch, Elsevier Inc., 1600 John F. Kennedy Blvd., Suite 1800, Philadelphia, PA 19103-2899

10. Owner (Do not leave blank. If the publication is owned by a corporation, give the name and address of the corporation immediately followed by the names and addresses of all stockholders owning or holding 1 percent or more of the total amount of stock. If not owned by a corporation, give the names and addresses of the individual owners. If owned by a partnership or other unincorporated firm, give its name and address as well as those of each individual owner. If the publication is published by a nonprofit organization, give its name and address.)

Full Name	Complete Mailing Address
Wholly owned subsidiary of	1600 John F. Kennedy Blvd. Ste. 1800
Reed/Elsevier, US holdings	Philadelphia, PA 19103-2899

11. Known Bondholders, Mortgagees, and Other Security Holders Owning or Holding 1 Percent or More of Total Amount of Bonds, Mortgages, or Other Securities. If none, check box ▸ ☐ None

Full Name	Complete Mailing Address
N/A	

12. Tax Status (For completion by nonprofit organizations authorized to mail at nonprofit rates) (Check one)
The purpose, function, and nonprofit status of this organization and the exempt status for federal income tax purposes:
☐ Has Not Changed During Preceding 12 Months
☐ Has Changed During Preceding 12 Months (Publisher must submit explanation of change with this statement)

PS Form 3526, August 2012 (Page 1 of 3 (Instructions Page 3)) PSN 7530-01-000-9931 PRIVACY NOTICE: See our Privacy policy in www.usps.com

---

13. Publication Title	14. Issue Date for Circulation Data Below
Heart Failure Clinics	July 2014

15. Extent and Nature of Circulation		Average No. Copies Each Issue During Preceding 12 Months	No. Copies of Single Issue Published Nearest to Filing Date
a. Total Number of Copies (Net press run)		183	208
b. Paid Circulation (By Mail and Outside the Mail)	(1) Mailed Outside-County Paid Subscriptions Stated on PS Form 3541. (Include paid distribution above nominal rate, advertiser's proof copies, and exchange copies)	52	45
	(2) Mailed In-County Paid Subscriptions Stated on PS Form 3541 (Include paid distribution above nominal rate, advertiser's proof copies, and exchange copies)		
	(3) Paid Distribution Outside the Mails Including Sales Through Dealers and Carriers, Street Vendors, Counter Sales, and Other Paid Distribution Outside USPS®	12	16
	(4) Paid Distribution by Other Classes Mailed Through the USPS (e.g. First-Class Mail®)		
c. Total Paid Distribution (Sum of 15b (1), (2), (3), and (4))	▸	64	61
d. Free or Nominal Rate Distribution (By Mail and Outside the Mail)	(1) Free or Nominal Rate Outside-County Copies Included on PS Form 3541		
	(2) Free or Nominal Rate In-County Copies Included on PS Form 3541		
	(3) Free or Nominal Rate Copies Mailed at Other Classes Through the USPS (e.g. First-Class Mail)		
	(4) Free or Nominal Rate Distribution Outside the Mail (Carriers or other means)		
e. Total Free or Nominal Rate Distribution (Sum of 15d (1), (2), (3) and (4))	▸	63	72
f. Total Distribution (Sum of 15c and 15e)	▸	127	133
g. Copies not Distributed (See instructions to publishers #4 (page #3))	▸	56	75
h. Total (Sum of 15f and g)	▸	183	208
i. Percent Paid (15c divided by 15f times 100)	▸	50.39%	45.86%

16. Total circulation includes electronic copies. Report circulation on PS Form 3526-X worksheet.

17. Publication of Statement of Ownership
If the publication is a general publication, publication of this statement is required. Will be printed in the October 2014 issue of this publication.

18. Signature and Title of Editor, Publisher, Business Manager, or Owner

[signature] Stephen R. Bushing – Inventory Distribution Coordinator

Date September 14, 2014

I certify that all information furnished on this form is true and complete. I understand that anyone who furnishes false or misleading information on this form or who omits material or information requested on the form may be subject to criminal sanctions (including fines and imprisonment) and/or civil sanctions (including civil penalties).

PS Form 3526, August 2012 (Page 2 of 3)

Moving?

Make sure your subscription moves with you!

To notify us of your new address, find your **Clinics Account Number** (located on your mailing label above your name), and contact customer service at:

Email: journalscustomerservice-usa@elsevier.com

800-654-2452 (subscribers in the U.S. & Canada)
314-447-8871 (subscribers outside of the U.S. & Canada)

Fax number: 314-447-8029

Elsevier Health Sciences Division
Subscription Customer Service
3251 Riverport Lane
Maryland Heights, MO 63043

*To ensure uninterrupted delivery of your subscription, please notify us at least 4 weeks in advance of move.

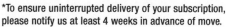

Printed and bound by CPI Group (UK) Ltd, Croydon, CR0 4YY

Printed and bound by CPI Group (UK) Ltd, Croydon, CR0 4YY

03/10/2024

01040377-0007